MIRACULOUS
HEALING

SUFFERING, DISEASE, AND CHRONIC PAIN WILL
QUICKLY DISAPPEAR

MIRACULOUS HEALING

SUFFERING, DISEASE, AND CHRONIC PAIN WILL

QUICKLY DISAPPEAR

RICHARD DORÉ

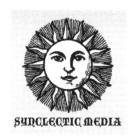

SYNCLECTIC MEDIA

Published by **Synclectic Media**
Seattle, Washington
www.synclectic.com

Publisher's Cataloging-in-Publication Data

Doré, Richard
  Miraculous Healing: Suffering, Disease, and Chronic Pain Will Quickly Disappear / Richard Doré. – 1st ed.
    p. cm. –
  Summary: Miraculous Healing shows how to use the power of mind to cure cancer and all other diseases. Simple and easy-to-use techniques are presented that can be learned in a few minutes. A new healing paradigm is being created and it will work for you.

  ISBN: 978-0615839950
  [1. Cancer—Alternative Treatment. 2. Cancer—Psychosomatic Aspects. 3. Stress Management.] I. Title.
  616.99'408—dc21   P-CIP

---

10 9 8 7 6 5 4 3 2 1

Ω
First Edition
Printed in the United States

This book is dedicated to the
end of suffering and disease as we know it.

10% of the publisher's proceeds from
Miraculous Healing will be donated to the
Amma Sri Karunamayi Jubilee Housing Project.
www.karunamayi.org

TABLE OF CONTENTS

INTRODUCTION

A Course in Miracles says, "All disease is of the mind." Notice it doesn't say *some* disease, it says *all* disease. This concept may seem foreign to you, especially if you think that modern medicine has the answers. You would think after spending billions of dollars on medical research, they would have discovered a cure for cancer and other life-threatening diseases. But, they still don't have a clue about how to cure cancer or any other major diseases. I can hear you say, "What about all of the marvelous advances in medicine we are being told about?" They are pure fiction.

If you look deeply into what has actually happened, and not just what the medical community is saying, you will find that the statistics tell a very different story. The survival rate for cancer patients in the last fifty years has changed very little; five percent is all. Those marvelous advances don't actually exist. Think about this: Medicine is a trillion dollar business in the United States alone. If they magically came up with a cure for cancer and other major diseases, it would put them out of business. So, what is the incentive to find a cure for cancer and other life-threatening diseases? There isn't one.

Is there a conspiracy to not find a cure? Frankly, I don't know. Modern medicine, like any bureaucracy, has developed a collective autocratic ego structure that resists change, at all costs. This is not unusual; all entrenched bureaucratic systems resist new ideas.

Change is abhorrent to ego, especially the collective ego; this is not a small matter. Ego's resistance can be as deadly as any disease. Throughout the book, I will talk a lot about how to cope with ego's resistance to change.

Over 500,000 people die of cancer every year in the United States alone. Worldwide, millions die every year for the same reason—collective ignorance. The real cause of disease is ignored by medicine. You may be wondering what makes me think I have the answer to curing disease. Well, I do, and it's right here in this book. The solution is so simple, it boggles the mind. Having said that, there are, of course, obstacles and pitfalls, but once you have the complete picture, you will know how to navigate around them.

I knew intuitively, when I read *The Course* many years ago, that when it said "All disease is of the mind," it was true. But, I also realized because of the culture's belief in medical science, I would have to wait for proof from the scientific community, before people would take what *The Course* said, seriously. Little did I know at the time, it would take a quarter of a century for biological research to validate what it says. *The Course* doesn't say how the mind creates disease or how to cure disease. I was on my own in that regard. Quite by accident, I developed a procedure for engaging the mind's ability to heal the body. With a little coaching, you can actually heal yourself. In fact, one of the key elements in the new healing paradigm being developed is taking responsibility for your own healing.

Recently, the scientific evidence I was waiting for showed up in the form of a book by Bruce Lipton, entitled, *The Biology of Belief.* He has a Ph.D. and is a cell biologist. His credentials are impeccable.

Most people would probably rather turn their health over to a doctor. But for the thousands of people who die of cancer every year in the United States who did just that, it didn't turn out very well. They suffered and died in agony, because of the barbaric procedures being used by modern medicine to treat cancer. Radiation and chemotherapy are still the mainstays for treating cancer. You can do your own research on the side effects and effectiveness of radiation and chemotherapy, by looking it up online. You will be stunned by what you find.

Medical treatments kill thousands of people every year. Of course, you never hear about it, because the medical community doesn't want you to know about them. The statistics around how many people die from cancer treatments are vague, especially around radiation and chemotherapy. Those procedures don't discriminate; they kill the healthy cells right along with the cancer cells. People don't always die from chemo and radiation, they die from complications. Chemo and radiation attack the organs of the body and can cause organ failure. So, the medical records show you died of liver or kidney failure.

Modern biology has caught up with *A Course in Miracles*, yet medicine still clings to its traditional approach to treating disease. How bad is it? Consider this. Almost all drugs treat symptoms only. They don't do anything about curing the disease. Despite the twentieth century's far-reaching discoveries about the mind, medicine has been reluctant to apply them to understanding cancer and other diseases.

The pharmaceutical companies continue to tout the fabulous benefits of the drugs they produce. They are some of the largest businesses in the world and they are very influential and profitable. The FDA is responsible for approving the drugs that pharmaceutical companies produce, but they have turned a blind eye to the fact that the drugs they approve don't actually cure disease. The system is corrupt.

The mind is divided into the conscious and unconscious (subconscious) minds. The conscious mind is the one you use to decide where you are going for lunch or to solve your day-to-day problems. It is the thinking mind. It can be monitored and controlled.

The unconscious mind is not so easily controlled. It is a major factor in disease. The content of the unconscious mind plays over and over and is largely outside of conscious control. It puts you on autopilot, for better or for worse. It stores the conditioning, beliefs, and thought forms that create what you experience, including disease. But, the unconscious mind can be accessed and the content changed. It is often dominated by compulsive negative thinking. Thought plays an important part in your body's chemistry. The role that mind and thought plays has been completely ignored by modern medical science, yet it is one of the major factors in disease. It is part of the disease equation.

A pivotal chapter is dedicated to clearing the unconscious mind of emotional trauma and thought forms. Most people are very reluctant to explore the content of their unconscious mind, but when they are diagnosed with a life-threatening disease like cancer, it then becomes a matter of survival. Obviously, at that point, you are faced with a choice. You can explore the depths of your unconscious mind—or not.

No one escapes some emotional trauma. As a child you didn't know how to deal with strong emotions, so you ignored and suppressed them. The residue from that trauma is still in your unconscious mind, stored as thought forms and energy patterns.

A young child has very slow brainwave activity. They are in Delta and Theta brainwaves until they are about six years old. A child in Delta or Theta brainwaves is unable to discriminate, so whatever they experience becomes their reality.

Your life is a direct reflection of the content of your unconscious mind and the beliefs contained within it. Beliefs can have positive or negative affects on your body chemistry. Disease is the result of the message being sent to your genes by your unconscious mind. Changing your mind can alter your genes. Contemporary biological research confirms that genes can be reprogrammed, even after they have mutated, and create disease.

Living in the twenty-first century, with all of the technology and modern conveniences, life should be easier. Still, for many, there is a gradual erosion of the quality of their lives. When you become ill, that erosion accelerates. Disease is a psychological event, so whatever has gone wrong in your body begins in your mind. What the mind creates, it can UN-create.

Your doctor will probably try to discourage you from the idea that disease is a product of the mind. The medical community is no closer to curing cancer and other life-threatening diseases than they were fifty years ago. Your doctor either doesn't know the truth, or he is in denial. To admit to the truth might put him out of business.

You may think you have come to this book by accident or sheer coincidence. Let me suggest it is the unseen hand of the universe, leading you to what you need to know in order to heal.

# # #

PART I

CREATING A NEW HEALING PARADIGM

CHAPTER ONE
THE POWER OF MIND

When your doctor gives up on you and sends you home to die, what are you going to do? Every year, here in the United States, over 500,000 people die from cancer. In spite of such a dire statistic, many people survive cancer through sheer determination and the mind's will to live.

There are 300 million people in the United States and almost half of them (139 million) have been diagnosed with some form of disease. Heart attacks are currently the number one killer in the U.S., with cancer following close behind. At the rate people are being diagnosed, cancer may soon surpass the annual death rate from heart disease. For many, it's no longer a question of whether you are going to get cancer, but when?

The idea of getting cancer strikes terror in the hearts of most people. Statistics show that one out of three women and one out of two men living in the U.S. will be faced with that diagnosis at some time in their lives. This prognosis is so terrorizing, because modern medicine doesn't have a clue what actually causes cancer or how to cure it. All they are really doing is attacking the symptoms.

Surgery is frequently used to treat cancer, and anyone who has had even a minor surgery can tell you how debilitating and traumatic it can be. It also weakens your immune system. Radiation and chemotherapy are the other traditional modalities used in treating cancer. Hair loss, abdominal pain, and even vomiting are the side effects of radiation and chemotherapy. Physical weakness and fatigue are additional consequences; they destroy healthy cells, along with the cancer cells. Harsh side effects is the good news. The bad news is that either having cancer, or being treated for it, can kill you.

A friend, who was a nurse, told me the story of her son's father who was suddenly diagnosed with cancer. He was hospitalized and the doctors thought that an aggressive treatment was the best way to tackle the disease. Within two weeks, he died. They believed he had lost his battle with cancer, but the autopsy showed he was cancer-free. What killed him? The treatment did. This is not unusual. These incidents are not often publicized because the medical community doesn't want you to know about them.

The number four killer in the U.S. is properly prescribed prescription drugs. Yes, I said properly prescribed drugs. It is reaching epidemic proportions. The news about the much heralded advances in modern medicine and cancer treatment is obscuring the facts. Perhaps you noticed I left out the number three killer of men, women, and children in the U.S. Well, here it is. It's the medical community in its entirety: hospitals, doctors, drugs, and all medical procedures. So, what in the world is going on? There is a crisis in modern medicine and we are not being told about it. Doctors and medicine occupy a place in our culture that nothing else does. They are held in the highest esteem, yet thousands of patients are dying as a direct result of medical treatment.

Recently, a United States Congress woman was shot in the head. She survived by getting to the hospital and going into surgery within 38 minutes from the time she arrived at the emergency room. It seems she will survive, but she has a long road of rehabilitation ahead of her and will likely never be the same. In addition, she had to survive being hospitalized. Of course, when you have a serious injury or have had a heart attack, you will want to get to a hospital emergency room as fast as you can. If you are alive when you reach a hospital emergency room, chances are good that you will survive. But other than that, being hospitalized is risky.

On a recent Larry King show on CNN, four doctors and cancer specialists were featured. They talked for an hour, but they didn't address how cancer is created (they don't know), except that lifestyle and stress contribute to the disease. They said people with cancer were living longer than they used to and that the survival rate has improved (only five percent in the past fifty years). Two things they talked about were how successful cancer treatment has become for prostate cancer, and that even though brain cancer is on the increase, there is little that can be done for it.

One of the doctors thought he might see the time when cancer would become a chronic disease, instead of traumatic and life-threatening, as it is now. Perhaps that is a better outcome than actually dying, but it is really surrendering to the disease.

You have cancer cells, pathogens, viruses, and bacteria in your body all of the time. When your immune system is suppressed, they can take over and cause disease. It is common knowledge that stress lowers the ability of the immune system to fight disease and that it is a contributing factor in the spread of cancer. Western societies breed stress like a swamp breeds mosquitoes. We all know that there is too much stress, but few do anything about it. What causes stress? Thought. Where does thought come from? The mind.

A Course in Miracles says that "All disease is of the mind." Notice, it doesn't say *some* disease, it says *all* disease. If you are a person who believes that only science has the answers, you may immediately want to discount what *The Course* says. After all, it is a spiritual text. Well, just hang in. What it says has been validated by science. It was published in 1976 by Helen Schucman and William Thetford, professors of medical psychology at Columbia University in New York City, NY. They were substantial figures in the medical community and were esteemed professionals, steeped in science and psychology. Schucman claimed the material for *The Course* was based on an inner voice she identified as Jesus. It came in the form of impressions, thoughts, and ideas which were written down. If you read it, you will not doubt its authenticity. At the time I read *The Course,* I was convinced that what it said about disease was true, but I had to wait decades for science to validate it. I didn't have the scientific evidence which many people want, until Bruce Lipton's book *The Biology of Belief* was published in 2005. He has a Ph.D. and is a cell biologist. He taught biology at the University of Wisconsin and Stanford Medical School. The book became a runaway bestseller. Since then, other studies and scientific evidence have validated that disease is a product of the mind.

The following is from an interview with Bruce Lipton and veteran science writer Jill Neimark:

"JN: How does subconscious programming influence the cell membrane?

"BL: When I have a thought, my mind sends out signals, in the form of growth factors, hormones, or other chemicals. Thoughts can also initiate rapid oscillations of nerve cells in unison, which creates a kind of field effect that influences other cells and neurons almost instantaneously. Now, what's interesting, and what I found out in my research at Stanford, is that your brain can veto what's going on in other places in your body. The signals sent out by your central nervous system actually override the function of cell membrane receptors that are responding to signals in their immediate environment. That means the brain can ultimately control the activity of tissues and organs. I believe that the most powerful information processing by the brain is in the domain of the subconscious (unconscious) and that it can shape tissue responses. These signals can actually influence the membrane to engage selected genes that then actively respond.

"When part of the brain senses stress, for example, it initiates a complex signal cascade that directs the body's cells to launch a protection response, particularly through a stress hormone called cortisol. Now, let's look at what happens to, say, a typical liver cell, which has receptors on its membrane that bind to cortisol. When it does this, the membrane sends information to the genes inside the nucleus of the cell to shut down their ability to break down a form of sugar, called glycogen. The genes stop doing this, and extra sugar is released into the blood. That sugar is used as energy to counter the stress. **This cascade could have been started by a belief that causes stress, even if it is a misperception.**"

For decades, there has been a lot of controversy around the placebo effect. Clinical trials show that forty percent of healing is the result of the placebo effect. Pharmaceutical companies are trying to limit its effect. Why? Because the potential for profit is nil. Many people get better when they "believe" that they are receiving medicine. Bruce Lipton calls it the "belief effect," to stress that our perceptions, whether they are accurate or inaccurate, impact cell behavior.

This is a powerful indication of the mind's ability to heal the body, and how belief can cause a positive or negative outcome. Modern biology has since caught up with *A Course in Miracles*. Quantum physics says the observer creates the observed, moment by moment. Quantum physics and the ancient spiritual teachings agree that you create what you experience. Why modern medicine has refused to look at the role mind plays in disease, is puzzling.

If you are like most people, you probably turn to your doctor when you are sick, hoping he will prescribe a pill to make your pain and suffering go away. The pain may go away, but ninety percent of all prescription drugs treat symptoms only. They absolutely don't cure disease. They may make you feel better, but they don't get to the root of the problem. So, sooner or later the disease will come back, usually sooner. That's what happens with most cancer patients. All prescription drugs have toxic side effects and as a rule, when there is a chronic problem, the dosage will need to be increased as time goes on. Often, they actually stop working completely, so the pain and discomfort return.

According to Kevin Trudeau, a leading consumer advocate, "Every non-prescription as well as prescription drugs increase the risk of disease." He goes on to say that "even over-the-counter non-prescription drugs, like aspirin and ibuprofen increase the risk of cancer."

Billions of dollars are spent treating cancer and other diseases. The actual amount is staggering, and exceeds 1.3 trillion dollars annually, in the U.S. alone. Many ad agencies receive most of their yearly revenue from pharmaceutical companies. Ten billion dollars are spent on advertising by pharmaceutical companies every year. If cancer and other life-threatening diseases were to magically disappear, many hospitals would close, doctors would be out of work, and pharmaceutical companies would go out of business.

Is there a conspiracy to not find a cure for the major diseases? Frankly, I don't think it is an out-right conspiracy, but it's easy to see that as long as cancer and other diseases remain incurable, doctors and employees of the pharmaceutical companies have job security.

You have probably heard many stories of people whose prognosis was dire, yet instead of becoming a victim, they dig in their heels and decide to live, despite the prognosis. How do they snatch victory from the jaws of defeat? Basically, they change their focus from defeat, to victory. They read books like this one that give them hope. They alter their diet, lifestyle, release stress, and, foremost, take responsibility for their own health.

There has been a lot of research on how emotions affect health. The conclusion is that the mind/body connection is a definite factor in illness. My job is to teach clients how to explore the mind/body connection to disease. Once they become aware of the connection for themselves, they begin to heal. Healing is achieved when you explore your own unconscious mind and become aware of the thought forms and beliefs that are creating your disease.

Everyone is up against ego's resistance to change. There are no exceptions. Ego *always* resists change. Ego is the guardian of the status quo and no matter how sick you become, it will resist change. Many people derive a sense of identity from being sick. If you have become chronically ill, it's likely you are identified with your illness and in this case, ego will staunchly defend its territory. Awareness is the key and once you become aware of your ego's resistance, it will begin to diminish. Resistance and negative thought forms cannot persist in the light of awareness.

The role stress plays in disease should not be underestimated. One of the best ways to eliminate stress is by practicing meditation. It increases intuition, creativity, and the connection to your Higher Nature. It has been practiced for centuries as part of many transformational disciplines. Recently, it has become widely accepted by the medical community as a tool for lowering blood pressure, enhancing the immune system, increasing mental ability, and accelerating healing.

Learning to meditate is a simple process. There are a lot of CDs available on how to meditate, and you will find a variety of styles to choose from. Or, you can take a class. They are usually inexpensive and are often free. If you don't already know how to meditate, make sure it's a class structured for beginners. Learning to meditate is like learning any other new skill; it will improve over time and with practice. If you are drawn to a certain style of meditating and it feels right to you, then it's appropriate. If you choose one that turns out to be a mismatch, then move on and try something else. You don't need to meditate more than ten to twenty minutes per day. Even five minutes can be very helpful.

There is a Buddhist meditation practice called Vipassana or "insight meditation," which is simple and easy to learn. Most meditation teachers will have you focus on something as you meditate because it helps you bypass chatter coming from the mind. In this style of meditation you focus on your breath.

The following excerpt is from the book entitled *The Art of Living*, by S.N. Goenka and William Hart. The language is a little arcane, but it is a good description on how to do Vipassana meditation:

"Respiration is an object of attention that is readily available to everyone, because we all breathe from the time of birth until the time of death. It is a universally accessible, object of meditation. To begin, sit down, assume a comfortable, upright posture, and close your eyes. Turning from the outer world to the world within, you find that the most prominent activity is your own breathing. So, you give attention to this object, the breath entering and leaving the nostrils.

"The effort is not to control the breath, but instead to remain conscious of it as it naturally is: long or short, heavy or light, rough or subtle. For as long as possible one fixes the attention on the breath, without allowing any distractions to break the chain of awareness.

"As meditators we find out at once how difficult this is. As soon as we try to keep the mind fixed on respiration, we begin to worry about a pain in the legs. As soon as we try to suppress all distracting thoughts, a thousand things jump into the mind: memories, plans, hopes, fears. One of these catches our attention, and after some time we realize that we have forgotten completely about breathing. We begin again with renewed determination, and again after a short time we realize that the mind has slipped away without our noticing."

The medical community seems to be oblivious to the fact that diet can affect genes and mitigate disease. It is actually more effective than many conventional treatments. A landmark Duke University study published in the August 1, 2003 issue of *Molecular Biology* found that an enriched environment can override genetic mutations in mice. In the experiment, one group of obese agouti mice received supplements available in health food stores: Folic acid, Vitamin B-12, Betaine, and Choline. In this case, diet was very effective at altering genes.

Cancer cells are the result of a gene gone wrong, or of a mutated gene. In some cases, lifestyle and dietary changes will actually eliminate cancer. Genetically, mice and rats are very similar to humans. It's clear that modern medicine has not yet caught up with *A Course in Miracles* or contemporary biological research.

A new healing paradigm is being created, where mind and self-awareness are the primary forces behind healing: You take responsibility for your own health. You recognize the role that ego plays in your disease. When allopathic medicine is used, you choose a doctor who takes a holistic approach. Alter diet, lifestyle, and release stress. Acknowledge the spiritual aspects of healing. The collective ego of the medical community will likely resist this new paradigm.

As you read along, you may notice that this book has a spiritual tone. If you are not used to the language, you may find it off-putting. But before you acquiesce to your ego's resistance to anything new (and that's exactly what it is), think about this: It is your ego in concert with your mind that creates disease. You now have a choice—to continue on, or surrender to ego's resistance to change.

CHAPTER TWO
A MIND DIVIDED

The mind is divided into the conscious and unconscious minds. The unconscious mind is indeed unconscious. It is simply a robotic-like device that puts you on autopilot. It has a definite link to ego; ego is the conscious and unconscious mind in motion.

The conscious mind is the volitional mind, the one you have control over. The conscious mind is the one you use when you decide to go to the grocery store before going to the post office, or whether to have lunch at McDonald's or Burger King. It can, in some cases, override the unconscious mind, but the unconscious mind is a lot more powerful. The conscious mind can process 4,000 bits of information a second. That seems powerful, doesn't it? Well, the unconscious mind can process 40,000 bits of information per second.

The unconscious mind is basically a computer and once it is programmed, it plays the same program over and over, playing the glitches right along with the good stuff. It has a mechanical nature. It can contain feelings and emotions, but they are not because of compassion or empathy. They are the result of previous input: garbage in, garbage out.

It is estimated that 98 percent of the time, you are responding to the information in your unconscious. Oddly enough, a lot of research has been done on how the unconscious mind works, but no one really knows where it is located. Most researchers think it's somewhere in the brain.

The brain is a receiver and, like a radio station, it receives a signal and then broadcasts the information it receives. It brings into focus the information and intelligence coming from the universe. Much of the esoteric information suggests the mind is a rotating field of energy outside of the body. Wisdom is certainly beyond the brain and its chemistry. The idea that mind is the result of chemistry is rather limited.

Science is not able to see the connection of the brain to the universe. There simply are no tools available to measure something as subtle as the energy and information coming to us from the universe. Wisdom, intuition, and creativity come from your Higher Nature, not from ego and brain. Many people in the Western cultures believe only in what comes from science. They tend to believe in a scientific approach where the hypothesis is validated over and over. The problem with this is that science is simply just another belief system and it functions like every other belief system. Beliefs are self-organizing or self-replicating. All biological and energetic structures are self-replicating. A belief will always appear to be true. All beliefs have the quality of drawing to them experiences that will verify and validate them. Everything you experience is the result of a self-replicating program or belief held in your unconscious mind.

What everyone seems to think is that humans have free will and choice. That's true, but it is seldom used, because you rely on the content of the unconscious mind. Multiple tasks are performed without thinking: taking a shower, brushing your teeth, cooking breakfast, walking, and many others. How many times have you driven along a highway and suddenly realized you had no idea how you got where you were? This is another example of how everyone relies on their unconscious mind.

The content of the unconscious mind is defended by ego with a tenacity seldom seen anywhere else in life. You can see this playing out on the daily talk shows, where the commentator defends his ideology to the point of absurdity. They are defending programs and beliefs that were formed earlier in life. The Roman Catholic Church takes the position that if they have the opportunity to educate, or should I say indoctrinate a child until he is six years old, he will always be a Catholic and for the most part, they are absolutely right.

From the time you are born, until you are six years old, your brainwaves are very slow. You are in Delta waves until two years of age and then Theta waves until you turn six. This slow brainwave activity probably reaches back into the womb. The fetus responds to external stimuli after about four and one-half months of development and begins to store emotions and feelings long before it is born.

The mother's chemistry and hormones transmit information to the fetus. This includes anger, fear, and other emotions. The brain is the first major organ to develop.

Brainwaves are divided into four parts; Delta is the slowest, followed by Theta, Alpha, and Beta. Beta is normal brainwave activity for children over twelve years of age and for adults. Brainwaves are measured in hertz, or cycles. Delta waves are 1-4 cycles per second, Theta waves are 4-7 cycles, Alpha waves are 7-13 cycles, and Beta waves are 13-60 cycles.

When you are in Delta waves, there is no filter, no way to resist any of the information that comes to you. Whatever you are exposed to goes directly into your unconscious mind and becomes your reality. Those slow brainwave states are the reason a child learns so much so quickly. Many children begin to play computer games at two and three years of age and vast amounts of information is learned. Most of the child's emotional development occurs in the first two or three years of his life, while in Delta and Theta brainwaves. Again, the mind has no filter during this time; therefore, it does not discriminate. It accepts the good information right along with the bad.

When a child is in Delta or Theta waves and there is emotional, sexual, or physical abuse, it becomes the child's reality. He will be abused for the rest of his life unless the content of the unconscious mind is changed. I will explain how to do that later. Thought, emotions, and feelings, can distort genes and create disease. A child always believes the abuse they experience is their fault; this subsequently turns to self-hatred and disdain for their body. This creates a situation where the unconscious mind may attack the body. One in three women is sexually abused. About the same percentage get cancer. This is no coincidence.

At two years of age, the child goes into Theta waves. This is still a state of openness and great receptivity. The imagination becomes very active. When a child is making mud pies, they are actually pies to him. When he is riding a broom pretending it's a horse, it is actually a horse.

These are the brainwave levels you experience when hypnotized. When you are hypnotized, the suggestions given by the hypnotist can make you quack like a duck, crow like a rooster, cluck like a chicken, and demonstrate incredible strength. Apparently, the suggestions cannot override your conscience or moral codes, but other than that, you can make a complete fool of yourself.

A friend of mine who worked in a Safeway supermarket had to learn a new system of codes for the produce, meat, and other items they sold at the checkout stand. She thought she would have a difficult time memorizing them, so she went to a hypnotist. He inserted a new belief into her unconscious mind that made it much easier to memorize the new codes. However, it's difficult to permanently override unconscious beliefs. The effects of hypnotism are usually temporary.

If you were sick a lot as a young child, sickness will likely become your reality, especially if it was reinforced by the attention you got from your parents. Biologists speak of genetic determination, that you are pre-disposed to illness because you inherit certain genes. It is much more likely that a particular genetic mutation was formed by the thoughts and emotions experienced while in Delta and Theta waves. According to Bruce Lipton, genes are not fixed. They respond readily to external stimuli and thoughts coming from the unconscious mind. Each gene carries the blueprint for over two thousand different proteins. Those proteins make up your DNA.

The following is from Bruce Lipton's book *The Biology of Belief:* "In this book I will draw the proverbial line in the sand. On one side of the line is a world defined by neo-Darwinism, which casts life as an unending war among battling, biochemical robots. On the other side of the line is the 'New Biology,' which casts life as a cooperative journey among powerful individuals who can program themselves to create joy-filled lives. When we cross that line and truly understand the New Biology, we will no longer fractiously debate the role of nurture and nature, because we will realize that the fully conscious mind trumps both nature and nurture. And, I believe we will also experience as profound a paradigmatic change to humanity as when a round-world reality was introduced to a flat-world civilization."

What activates genes? The answer was put forth in 1990, in a paper entitled, *Metaphors and the Role of Genes and Development,* by H. F. Nijhout. He presents evidence that the belief that genes control biology has been repeated for such a long time, scientists have forgotten it is a hypothesis. The idea that genes control biology has never been proven, and has been undermined by the latest scientific research. Genetic control has become a belief in our culture. You want to believe that genetic manipulators can cure disease and that, while they are at it, can create super humans. Lipton says that trauma, toxins, thought, and the unconscious mind, control genes and determine whether you have good health or disease.

What gets suppressed in your unconscious mind as an unborn child? As a fetus or an infant, you suppress feelings and emotions. You don't suppress thoughts or even concepts. Much of the information you acquire and suppress comes from the mother's chemistry. Thoughts create chemistry and hormones, which become feelings and emotions.

A child, long before he can cognize, learns that some emotions and feelings cannot be expressed in his family. All families restrict certain emotions and feelings. The child realizes if he is to survive, he must not express those emotions and feelings.

Anger is off limits in some families, and in many, you can't express your anger without feeling like you will be severely punished. At least that's the way the child often sees it. There is a direct correlation between suppressed anger and heart problems, and there is a relationship between fear and cancer. Long-term fear weakens the immune system.

The following is from Deb Shapiro's book, *Your Body Speaks Your Mind: Decoding the Emotional, Psychological and Spiritual Message that Underlies Illness:* "There are also some well-researched characteristics of the cancer personality as one that includes a suppression of strong emotions, particularly anger and passion; lack of assertiveness, especially in expressing your own needs; stoicism; avoidance of conflict; and appearance of incest. Obviously, not all cancer patients have these characteristics, for cancer is nothing if not multifaceted and indiscriminant. There is undoubtedly a mystery factor involved here. But cancer has lessons for us all about our attitudes toward each other, about accepting and loving unconditionally, and especially about loving ourselves. Many cancer survivors have spoken about how their healing came as they began to honor themselves more deeply.

"More especially, cancer gives you the chance to re-evaluate, to take stock and be more honest about your feelings, and to clarify your priorities. Just as negative or repressed emotions compromise the immune system, so research (such as in Stanford) has shown that therapy—particularly group therapy, where feelings can be released in a caring environment with the support of others—can make a huge difference to the healing process. Talking and feeling safe enable you to find those lost and alienated parts of yourself, to give them life and bring them back into the whole.

"Exploring the function of the part of the body involved will help you deepen your understanding. It is also essential to strengthen the immune system, which means strengthening the desire to live. Those who develop a fighting spirit, mental resilience, and vigor, and who do not reject themselves, appear to have a greater survival rate. This is about developing an 'I want to live' attitude."

In order to restore health, you must become your own healer. I'm not suggesting you stop seeing your doctor or taking medication, but *you* are ultimately responsible for your own healing.

The concept that everything is energy was first put forth by Dr. Albert Einstein, early in the twentieth century in his famous equation $E=mc^2$. Why is this important? Because you are a complex structure of overlapping fields of energy and the only way to create permanent change is to raise the frequency of those fields. Those energy fields make you human and conscious; they create self awareness, intuition, creativity, and perception. Only humans have those qualities and the ability to choose how they are going to use them.

The following is from Bruce Lipton's book, *The Biology of Belief:* "The behavior of energy waves is important for biomedicine because vibrational frequencies can alter the physical and chemical properties of an atom as surely as physical signals like histamine and estrogen. Because atoms are in constant motion, which you can measure by their vibration, they create wave patterns similar to the expanding ripples from thrown pebbles. Each atom is unique because the distribution of its negative and positive charges, coupled with its spin rate, generates a specific vibration or frequency pattern (Oschman 2000)."

As you acknowledge and explore the idea that you are essentially an energy structure, you will open to the possibility that you can intentionally raise the frequency of your energy field. An interesting fact is that energy cannot be either created or destroyed. It can only be transformed. That said, as you begin to raise the frequencies of who you are, you will actually change your energy signature. Your conscious and unconscious minds are energy structures.

Negative thoughts form an energy pattern in your unconscious mind. Those thought forms alter your body chemistry and hormones and create disease. Those thought forms can be transmuted. No amount of will or positive suggestion will affect them. The transformative element is the energy of self-awareness.

Because energy is always moving in order to be physically healthy, your energies must flow effortlessly. When you suppress feelings and emotions, you are blocking the flow of energy in your body. You are very much like a steam boiler. You must have a release valve that allows the energy to flow freely, or chaos will occur in your field. Your release valve is your awareness.

Trying to control your feelings and emotions will diminish your energy flow. Energy, like water, needs to move or it becomes stagnant and toxic. Emotion is actually intense thought. The purpose of emotions is to trigger a release, so the energy can begin to flow. When an emotion is not totally expressed, it leaves a residue. The left over energy creates a pattern in your field. Those stagnant energies then become a harbinger for disease.

Anger is actually energy and it wants to move. Anger is a boundary defense and whenever your boundaries are violated, you become angry. If you are not able to express your anger, it accumulates. When there is abuse of any kind, there is anger. The boundaries of an abused child are violated, time and time again. If the child doesn't express his anger, he will turn it inward and create self-hatred. Anger is often suppressed to the point where the person is totally unaware of his anger. When it surfaces, it can be devastating to the individual and to others around them. A sign of suppressed anger is depression. As you read this, it may trigger your own suppressed anger. You may simply feel a little agitated at first; that agitation is your anger bubbling to the surface. Allow yourself to express it, or the pressure will keep on building.

Energy follows thought. Thoughts can have a profound affect on cells. Negative thoughts create low, slow frequencies which encourage the growth of disease. Low frequencies are often expressed in the body as low pH; cancer and other diseases thrive in acidic conditions. In Norman Cousins' bestselling classic *The Anatomy of an Illness,* he says that laughter is a great antidote for diseases. Laughter raises your frequencies, which encourages healing.

There are many hands-on energy healing practices. The most well known is Reiki. They are all supposed to heal or cure disease, but it has been my experience that most hands-on healing practitioners are not very successful. In order for a practitioner to be successful, they must clear their own field and unconscious mind of negative patterns, and be able to hold and transmit a very high frequency; few can do that. The higher the frequency, the more conscious it is. It is actually consciousness/awareness that does the healing. It's incredibly difficult to put consciousness into words and describe it. But, I will try with this simple statement: It is the essence of God. The higher the frequency, the more essence it contains.

Thought forms and beliefs are not indestructible. The Law of Entropy states that higher frequencies transmute lower frequencies; this is one of the keys to curing disease. Once the energy of a cell is raised, it can no longer support disease.

One of the reasons drugs are not effective and have such harsh side effects is that they are synthesized chemical structures and have a low frequency. Natural remedies tend to have a higher frequency and are a lot less toxic. In many cases, they are non-toxic. Edgar Cayce, the turn-of-the-twentieth century mystic and healer, said this: "Remember, thoughts are things and their contents run deep."

# # #

CHAPTER THREE
A LIFE SAVER

Every day 4,000 people in the United States are diagnosed with cancer. If you fit the profile of a person who is likely to get cancer, a little prevention will help enormously. The profile of a person who gets cancer is simply a person with a lot of stress, and is unwilling or unable to express emotions and feelings. If you have suppressed a lot of fear, as almost everyone has, this is especially true for you.

It is difficult for many people to express fear or anger, but it can actually be a life saver when these emotions *are* expressed. When humans first began to appear on earth, fear was very useful, because large carnivores saw humans as a food source and easy to prey upon. But, with their large brains and superior intellect, humans began to turn the tide on carnivores, and became the hunters. But superior intellect or not, the medical community still ignores the real cause of cancer and other diseases.

The following is from Dr. Bernie Siegel's book, *Love, Medicine & Miracles:* "Despite the twentieth century's far-reaching discoveries about the mind, medicine has been strangely reluctant to apply them to a better understanding of cancer. Elida Evans, a student of Carl Jung, paved the way in 1926 with her *Psychological Study of Cancer,* but it went almost completely ignored. The copy I came across in the Yale Medical Library in the mid-1970s had been borrowed only six times in fifty years. The book clearly spells out the cancer risk incurred by the personality type for whom life's meaning comes entirely from people or things outside the self. When that connection is disrupted, illness follows, Evans concluded. Cancer is a symbol, as most illness is, of something going wrong in the patient's life, a warning to him to take another road."

So where has the medical community been for the past 86 years? The answer is—out to lunch! Cells have brains and when it comes to knowing when to retreat or move forward and multiply, they are plenty smart. Everyone and everything, right down to the smallest cell, wants to expand and grow. This determination to multiply is reflected in the over-population of the planet. It is leading to a lack of available resources. The air is barely breathable in many large cities, especially in China. The oceans are being over fished. Even clean drinking water isn't available in many areas of the world. The earth's top soil is being depleted. The prognosis for the earth and humans is dire. There is a lot we can do to begin to repair the damage, but first you must begin with yourself—physically, emotionally, and spiritually.

Interestingly, the over-population and destruction of the planet, mirrors what is occurring within humanity. In spite of this dire scenario, some religions still promote large families and go so far as to suggest that birth control is a sin and is forbidden. One of my favorite authors and teachers, Eckhart Tolle, says that humans are "dangerously insane." He could be right. Over one hundred million people were killed in wars during the twentieth century. If that's not insanity, what is?

Fear is almost always a major issue in cancer, and it has a number of negative impacts on your biology. Cells actually contract in the face of fear. Growth and healing are arrested when you are fearful. One of the reasons for this is that the blood supply goes to your extremities when you are in the flight mode. In the process, the immune system is suppressed. Your ability to fight cancer and other illnesses is reduced.

When you suppress your emotions and feelings, you are actually suppressing your entire energy system, limiting the flow of energy throughout your body. The flow of energy is extremely complicated and modern medicine knows nothing about it.

The primary energy systems of the human body are called chakras. Chakra is a Sanskrit word that means "wheel." When your chakras are balanced, you are healthy and vibrant, but when one or more of them becomes blocked or out of balance, you will become stressed and experience physical and emotional dysfunction. When a chakra is out of balance and its energy isn't flowing properly, the organs associated with it will not function as they should and become subject to disease.

There are seven major chakras. The three lower chakras are connected to the earth and are involved with emotions and feelings. The four upper chakras are connected to your higher energies and they function together as one system. The following describes the seven major chakras:

Root Chakra—Sanskrit name—Muladhara. The root chakra is located at the tip of the spine where the coccyx is located. It connects you to the earth. Many people are disconnected from the planet because their root chakra is distorted or out of balance. You are a child of the earth and you need the nourishing energy it provides.

The emotional issues associated with the root chakra are survival, betrayal, and abandonment. They are stored in the root chakra. When you store issues in your chakras, it throws them out of balance and limits the ability of the chakras to nourish the organs they are identified with. If you were abused as a child, you will have survival and betrayal issues stored in your first chakra. You will probably be ungrounded and disconnected from the earth and you will find it hard to concentrate and stay focused.

The first chakra is important because of its influence on your psychology. Mainstream psychologists and psychiatrists don't recognize the root chakra's importance in mental health. In fact, most of them don't even know it exists. In order to heal emotional trauma, the root chakra must be cleared and reconnected to the earth, or the therapy will be unsuccessful. This is especially true where there is severe trauma, like when there is emotional and physical abuse.

The psychiatric community tries to overcome their ignorance by prescribing drugs, and as I said earlier, ninety percent of drugs treat symptoms, but 100 percent of those drugs have toxic side effects and many have a debilitating effect on brainwave activity.

The root chakra is associated with the adrenals, colon, bones, prostate, and even your fingernails.

Sacral Chakra—Sanskrit name—Svanhisthana is located about two and one-half inches below the navel. It is related to sexuality, relationships, and creativity. Creativity is the hallmark of being human. When this chakra is out of balance it impairs creativity. When your boundaries are not respected as a child, the anger will be stored in the sacral chakra. The issues you have around sexuality and your relationships will impact this chakra.

The sacral chakra is associated with sex organs, kidneys, and the bladder.

Solar Plexus Chakra—Sanskrit name— Manipura. This chakra is located at the base of the sternum, where the solar plexus is located. It deals with your personal power, self-esteem, action, and vitality. Almost everyone has personal power issues, because as a child, you were not allowed to totally express your personal will and feelings. This is a tricky parental issue, because the child must learn to respect others, yet be allowed to express their personal will and feelings appropriately. If parents are not successful at this, their children are disempowered.

This chakra is associated with the liver, digestive system, spleen, and nervous system.

When the solar plexus chakra is blocked, your personal influence and will power become limited. You will also be relegated to a subordinate position with your peers and those you work with. And, if *that* weren't enough, your upper chakras will not function properly. The entire system works as one unit and in order to function properly, the energy must flow from the lower chakras through the upper chakras.

Heart Chakra—Sanskrit name—Anahata. The heart chakra is located in the center of the chest and is associated with love, compassion, forgiveness, and healing. The heart center is one of the master centers and is associated with the highest qualities of what it means to be human. The joy and bliss that occurs when the heart center opens, is like nothing I have experienced in any other way. The heart is the receptor of love, joy, and even prosperity. Stress, fear, anger, and frustration, tend to close the heart center and make you less receptive to well-being. When a child does not receive enough love, he or she will revert back to the solar plexus chakra and try to get what he wants through personal will.

The heart center is associated with the physical heart, blood, and immune system, the skin, upper back, and lungs.

Throat Chakra—Sanskrit name—Vishuddha. This chakra controls self-expression, confidence, wisdom, and supernatural abilities; it is where the Adam's apple is located. I seem to have a hyperactive throat chakra and any time I do a lot of meditation, my throat chakra blows wide open and I become difficult to be around. I cannot keep from telling people what I see in them. All of us are speaking half truths and sometimes even *less* than that, so when I hear those lies, I have to speak about it. Ordinarily, I am quite political and try not to offend other people, but when my throat chakra has blown open—watch out! *No one* around me is safe! The throat chakra and the second chakra are linked together. You express your creativity through your throat chakra.

The throat chakra is associated with the thyroid, jaw, neck, and larynx.

Third Eye Chakra—Sanskrit name—Ajna. The third eye, or brow chakra, is located just above and between the eyebrows. It is related to inner vision, intuition, imagination, extrasensory perception, and psychic abilities. Many of the yoga traditions focus on the activation of this chakra, because you are said to be "enlightened" when your third eye opens and you can see God.

Organs associated with the third eye are the pituitary, left hemisphere of the brain, left eye, nose, sinuses, and nervous system.

Crown Chakra—Sanskrit name—Sahasrara. The crown chakra is located at the top of the head. It is associated with unity, universal wisdom, purpose, and consciousness. It is activated when you clear all of your other chakras.

Organs associated with the crown chakra are the pineal, cerebrum, right hemisphere of the brain, nervous system, and right eye. It is also associated with enlightenment.

When any of the seven chakras become out of balance, your well-being is impaired. Your chakras can be balanced by simply focusing on them during your meditations. Spending a minute or two focused on a particular chakra will rebalance its energy. In order for your chakras to remain balanced, you need to clear the issues stored in them.

There are many energy practices that will balance your chakras. Chi Gong, Kundalini Yoga, and yoga exercises are some I recommend. There are books, CDs, and DVDs available in stores or online that provide tools for clearing and balancing your chakras.

There is a chakra test on The Web; just Google the words chakra test. It will tell you if your chakras are out of balance. The test only takes about ten minutes and is very accurate. Does your doctor know enough about these energy systems to suggest that you do yoga exercises to balance your chakras? Probably not. The various yoga systems have been around for thousands of years. In the 60s, as a result of the hypocrisy of Western cultures, the youth revolted. During this time period, many of the Eastern teachings were brought to the West, yet they are still mostly ignored by the mainstream Western cultures. As these ancient teachings came to the West, they were integrated into Western spiritual thought, and to a lesser degree, contemporary psychology. Alternative therapies and energy practices began to emerge.

The distortion in your chakras and energy field is the result of thought. If a thought doesn't bring you peace, it will have a negative influence on your energies. A thought that is fear or anger-based, needs to be transmuted before it creates a downward emotional spiral that ends in hopelessness and despair; they are very contracted states. Integration, balance, and wholeness are your natural states. When you are in those states, there is a natural clarity to your thinking. There are a number of simple techniques available, to assist in monitoring and controlling your thinking. They will be talked about later.

One of the most contracted states you can experience is depression; it is suppressed anger. Suppressed anger can lead to heart attacks. It can also lead to liver disease. It's no coincidence that the Chinese word for liver and anger are the same. Liver transplants are often necessary, because people do not know how to cope with their anger. It would simply be a lot easier to learn to express your anger. The body rejects transplanted organs. In order to prevent rejection, the doctor will prescribe stress hormones that will depress your already weakened immune system. Cancer is often the result of a weak immune system.

The following is from Web MD, reviewed by Robert J. Bryg, MD: "If a caller upsets you, do you hurl the phone across the room? Do you curse and blast the horn furiously if the driver in front of you takes three seconds to notice the green light? An angry temperament can hurt more than relationships—anger and heart disease may go hand in hand, according to experts."

"You're talking about people who seem to experience high levels of anger very frequently," says Laura Kubzansky, PhD, MPH, an assistant professor at the Harvard School of Public Health who has studied the role of stress and emotion on cardiovascular disease.

"But explosive people who throw things or scream at others may be at greater risk, as well as those who harbor suppressed rage," she says. "Either end of the continuum is problematic."

"Scientists don't all agree that anger plays a role in heart disease, she says. "But many studies have suggested a significant link." 'I think the case is strong," Kubzansky says.

"For example, one large study published in *Circulation* in 2000, found that among 12,986 middle-aged African-American and white men and women, those who rated high in traits such as anger—but had normal blood pressure—were more prone to coronary artery disease (CAD) or heart attack. In fact, the angriest people faced roughly twice the risk of CAD and almost three times the risk of heart attack compared to subjects with the lowest levels of anger."

A client of mine who had her spleen removed, had an extremely weakened immune system. When she asked her doctor how to strengthen her immune system, he said he didn't know how. Actually, there are many supplements available which will enhance your immune function. Doctors receive minimal training in nutrition. The pharmaceutical companies don't produce natural remedies, because they can't patent them. In other words, there is a lot more profit in synthetic drugs.

Thoughts are energy structures. Once a thought enters your unconscious mind, it will attach to similar thoughts and begin creating a thought form. Studies show that about 70 to 75 percent of all thoughts are negative. It's probably closer to 95 percent for many people. There are always negative thought forms in your unconscious mind when there is disease. Those forms eagerly attract similar energies. What's at work here is resonance and what some call the Law of Attraction, which means like attracts unto itself. Birds of a feather, flock together, is another way of saying the same thing. Thought forms can become huge and create chaos in your unconscious mind. They can dominate your life as they do with many compulsive mental issues: paranoia, schizophrenia, bipolar, depression, and others. The psychiatric community finds it easier to prescribe drugs for those conditions, but often they don't work and the side effects can be horrific. If the underlying emotional issues are not cleared, disease is the likely outcome.

If you are taking drugs for mental issues and are benefiting from them, you are not being advised to stop taking them. With most medications, however, the longer you are on them, the more you will have to take. Any time a drug stops working, you need to look at the issues that are causing the disease.

If you have become chronically ill, your ego will see this as your reality and it will resist change, no matter how sick you are. Your illness, whether mental or physical, is only part of the problem. Ego's resistance to change is a bigger obstacle. You can learn to cope with your resistance, and once you become aware of how it works, it will begin to diminish. Resistance cannot persist in the light of awareness. The universe is self-healing and will create wellness and balance whenever it can. But without self-awareness, nothing will happen.

A Course in Miracles says, "You have the disease because you value it." This may be a little hard to swallow, but it is true. I have sinus infections from time-to-time and I can always trace them back to feeling overwhelmed. The infection takes me out of the feeling of being overwhelmed and creates a distraction. Children often get sick to get attention from their parents; it's a way of getting love.

In working with clients, the first step is to discover the underlying reason for the disease. One of my clients, Joan, had a severe blood disease and had been hospitalized for treatment. It was nearly fatal. During a session, she discovered it was a way of not dealing with her husband and not standing up for herself.

Joan's husband was emotionally abusive and controlling. He listened to her phone calls. When she went into her bedroom and closed the door (she had her own bedroom), he would barge in without knocking. He wouldn't let her out of his sight for more than a few minutes. During forty years of marriage, she never had any privacy. The house she lived in had become a prison, but she never complained or fought back. Her boundaries were constantly violated, but she never expressed her anger. Instead, she turned her anger inward and became ill. As a child, her mother was constantly critical and complained about her behavior. Joan never got what she wanted. When her mother asked her what she wanted, she always gave her something else. If Joan wanted a Barbie doll to play with, her mother would give her a panda bear. If that happened once or even twice, it wouldn't matter so much, but it happened constantly. She grew up with the expectation of never getting what she desired and not being able to ask for what she wanted. And, whenever Joan complained, her mother scolded her and withheld love from her. Throughout her life, she attracted people to her who were just like her mother. Joan's response to her husband was very self-destructive and it almost killed her.

There is no way you can change the outer world. You have already tried that with your spouse, relationship, children, friends, and associates and you have been totally unsuccessful. You have to change your own inner programming before you can stop attracting what you don't want into your life. But nothing will change if you continue to accept the world view that you are a victim of external circumstances.

Perhaps you have heard this before, that you create your own reality and life experiences. So, why are you hearing it again? This is because as they say, you didn't get it when you heard it before. You may have given it lip service, you may even have nodded your head in agreement, but you are still not living your life as though you are the only one responsible for it. No matter how many doctors you see, you are responsible for your own health and until you take responsibility, you will not get well.

I made my initial exploration into this concept over thirty years ago, and even now, every once in awhile, I catch myself playing the "blame game." It takes persistence to change your beliefs. You may find it perplexing and difficult to actually live this way, but that's only because your ego doesn't want to accept this idea as being true. It's like a bulldog. Once it bites into something, it doesn't want to let go of it. There is also a collective belief in victimization at work here; it permeates the energy of the culture and the world at large. Can you imagine how the world would look if governments and people took full responsibility for their actions and for what they experience? Once you really get this, the door will open for accelerated integration and healing.

The universe wants you to regain authority over your life. It may be hard to swallow—that you, and *only* you are the one who creates everything you experience, including disease. Here is the good news. Because you create it, you have the power to UN-create it and heal. What I am saying to you is also supported by quantum physics. John Wheeler, a renowned quantum physicist, says, "There is no out there, out there." Everything you experience comes from within you and is a reflection of your inner landscape.

How do you know what your inner programming looks like? Just take a look at what you are experiencing. It is all a reflection of the beliefs stored in your unconscious mind. All of the issues in your life, your relationships, and even those chance encounters that are so annoying, are reflections of what you are harboring in your unconscious mind.

In order to heal, you need to change your lifestyle, reduce stress, get more exercise, and change your diet. In addition, you must clear your unconscious mind of negative conditioning (this is the most important step), beliefs, and thought forms. If you are one of the lucky ones who are not already ill, this same approach will prevent you from becoming a statistic.

# # #

CHAPTER FOUR
INNER RESOURCES

One of Buddha's most well-known statements is, "Life is suffering." Life is a struggle for most, and it gets even *more* difficult when you are sick. The human dilemma is that we are greatly influenced, and even controlled, by compulsive thinking. Everybody is thinking all of the time and those thoughts are, as you know, at least 75 percent negative. Remember, energy follows thought. Negative thoughts cause your energies to contract and produce lower frequencies, allowing disease to easily take hold. Thought plays a major role in your body chemistry and the amount of stress you experience. Monitoring your thoughts will decrease stress and diminish their impact on your body's chemistry.

Most dysfunctional behavior is the result of ego's resistance to change, and avoiding the old, repressed material in your unconscious mind. Making significant changes requires learning how to cope with your ego's resistance and allowing those old, suppressed feelings and memories to arise. You may feel a strong repulsion toward allowing them to come up. What is really going on is an old childhood program is playing, that says you will be punished, or even killed, if you let those feelings surface and express them. That belief is preventing you from going within your unconscious mind and clearing those issues. All emotions, including the anger that wasn't expressed as a child, are still in your energies; they will create physical symptoms and disease. Those unexpressed feelings become energetic patterns and thought forms in your unconscious mind. They actually lower the frequencies of your intellect and impede your creativity.

Thoughts are like fertilizer to the unconscious mind. They grow the already existing thought forms, which lead to even more compulsive thinking. Emotions and feelings can lie dormant for a long time, and just as you think your life has begun to flow effortlessly, you find those programs are not entirely dormant.

Self-awareness is the key to healing. Often, people try to allow just enough awareness into their lives so they can get from one point to another. Guarded awareness, it might be called. Limiting what you experience disconnects you from the wisdom of the universe.

If you allow your awareness to expand, you will become aware of your inner wisdom and Higher Nature. Your Higher Nature knows more about healing your life than you or your doctor could ever know, because it exists beyond polarity. It resides outside of time and space. Those gut feelings that have guided you in the past, are your inner wisdom communicating with you. It will lead you to what you need to know and experience in order to heal, just as it has led you here.

Most, if not all, conditioning and beliefs are fear-based and negative. Ego is fear-based. As a child, you could have been taught truth, but chances are you weren't. Your parents could have been unconditional in their love toward you, but they probably were not. They could have taught you that you are being supported by a loving and caring universe that sees you and everyone else as special, but they probably didn't. You could have been taught that you are safe, secure, and will always be protected, that life is a joyous creation, but you probably weren't. Most of us were taught that danger and sickness are lurking just around the corner. And of course, if that's what you believe, then that's exactly what you will experience.

Most people see the world through beliefs that look like these: the only thing that is real is what I can see, feel, touch, smell, or hear. We are all victims of circumstances and bad luck. Others are out to take advantage of us. No one is secure. Life is threatening and unpredictable. Life is a struggle and there's no way out. I have to work hard to get what I want. (Usually, this means you have to work your fingers to the bone.) No matter *how* hard I work, I never seem to get ahead. Life is out of control and there is nothing anyone can do about it. I'll never get what I want because I'm too old, too fat, too skinny, too tall, too short, too ugly, or I don't have enough education to get ahead. And here is the kicker, the one that is the most debilitating and is the real reason for your disease: there is never enough love for me. Disease is the result of a broken heart. Your essence is love, but you are not aware of it because of negative conditioning. With beliefs like those, it will be very difficult to trust the wisdom of the universe and your Higher Nature to heal you.

Where does all that emotional pain and suffering come from? It comes from your "pain body," an energetic structure that has split off from your total energies and has taken on a life of its own. It contains fear, anger, and emotional issues that are kept alive by energy coming from others. In other words, your own fear and anger are being reflected back to you from another pain body; that's how it feeds itself.

The pain body forms, because every time you become emotional and experience fear, anger, and other issues, some of the energies are suppressed, usually most of them. Energy keeps building up as the pain body continues to feed off other people's emotions and energy. As a result, you will find yourself de-volving rather than e-volving, as time passes and you grow older. As you de-volve, you become more likely to attract sickness.

In order to clear pain body issues, you need to feel, embrace, and acknowledge them as they come up; it can be unpleasant as they surface. Since ego seeks pleasure and avoids pain, it prefers to keep them under wraps. When you are conscious and aware of your issues as they arise, you can easily clear them. Just call in your Higher Nature to clear them for you. I usually start by clearing patterns on my own. If my resistance is particularly strong, I'll work with someone I trust who can assist me in releasing the resistance and issues. I may even work with a therapist. Your pain body fights to survive. Like the Nile crocodile, it can go for a long time without eating, but sooner or later your pain body will come out to feed. If it's been deprived of food for a considerable length of time, it will surface with a ravenous appetite and will create a lot of chaos and emotional pain in the process. Of course, the turmoil and pain will look like it is coming from someone else, but it's not; your issues are being mirrored back to you. At this point, you can choose to dive into them and clear them, or deny and suppress them.

You may have a spouse or a partner who has been supportive. On the surface, the relationship has been free of conflict, and then all of a sudden, you find yourself in a war, way out of proportion to events. You rage, curse, throw things, fight, and argue over what your partner has done to you. What has happened is that your pain body has come out to feed. It looks like the conflict is caused by what someone else has said or done to you. That's exactly what your pain body wanted. Their response has given it permission to "let it all hang out," and since it needs others to feed off, you will choose a relationship that resonates with your emotional issues.

Many years ago, *my* pain body came out to feed. This wasn't the first time, but it was one of the most explosive. I had been experiencing severe financial difficulties and though I handled the emotions pretty well on the *outside,* I was seething beneath the surface. I wasn't aware of just how much emotion and anger were in my pain body.

It was a warm June evening and I was having dinner with my wife and daughter, who was about fourteen at the time. I had downed a couple of beers before dinner, so the stage was being set for what was about to happen. My wife and daughter started one of their "let's gang up on Dad" scenarios, for what had happened to us financially. I felt like I had done the best I could at the time, but it clearly wasn't good enough for them.

My wife and daughter were poking a sharp stick into the eye of a very large beast, which was about to surface and scare the hell out of them. Before I knew it, my rage erupted and I felt like I wanted to kill someone. It wasn't *completely* the result of my current financial problems; a lot of the anger was about being abused as a child. While I wasn't physically abusive during this incident, my wife told me later that I had thrown a large salad bowl at her. My daughter quickly disappeared into her bedroom and locked the door. I slammed the front door as I left the house, raging like a bull that had just been stabbed by a matador. That incident was the beginning of the end of my marriage. A few months later, I joined a group where I was able to safely express my anger.

We've all seen stories on television like this, where one family member flies into a rage and kills another, sometimes killing the entire family. It often happens during stressful times, like around Christmas. This scenario is a result of suppressing anger and saying no to feelings. Saying no makes your ego feel stronger and strengthens its sense of control. It's the most powerful stance it can take. Sooner or later, you will pay the price for saying no. Often, the trapped energy will become so toxic that it will create disease, like heart attacks, cancer, arthritis, diabetes, and others. Saying no to your feelings simply creates more stress.

All addictions are a way of trying to fill a void that was created during childhood. Alcohol, drugs, and food addictions are simply an attempt to numb the pain body, however it never works. Ego wants to avoid the pain as long as possible, but in doing so, your emotional issues and toxic energies will keep adding layer upon layer, like an onion. Those energies will keep right on building—until they explode!

Remember, Buddha said that life is suffering, but he didn't leave us without an answer to that dilemma. He said the way out of suffering is to look deeply *within* the suffering. Of course, nobody wants to look at the reason for their suffering. It's just too scary, or at least that's the way it seems.

Control is what your ego thinks it needs for survival. Ego is simply a program set in motion by conditioning. You are on autopilot because of it and even if you are flying into a mountain, and about to crash, your ego will not alter its course.

How do you know what your conditioning and beliefs are? Again, they are reflected back to you by others and by the circumstances of your life. If a lot of your friends have cancer or other diseases, they are warning you of the danger ahead if you don't make some changes. The most annoying people in your life, the ones who really piss you off, are the most *like* you. You don't like hearing this, but it is true.

Robert was describing someone he works with as a real jerk—someone really despicable. So, I told him that what he was seeing was a reflection, that there was something about himself being reflected back to him that he was not aware of.

"I'm a jerk," he commented.

"No," I replied.

His issue was that women always betray him. It was a belief he had developed as a child, yet at age fifty, it was still showing up in his life. Everyone has issues they have denied as a child, stuck in their unconscious mind. They are being reflected back to you in your relationships.

Our entire social structure is organized to keep you powerless. It is set up to keep you distracted from self-awareness to the point where hardly anyone is aware of what would be the most fulfilling thing they could accomplish. The major culprits are the advertising media and the TV programs that we are all exposed to. Some of the most popular are talk shows, where the hosts express their opinions and ideology. They talk incessantly about how we are all victims of circumstances beyond our control. And, no matter what is being experienced, it is always someone else's fault.

Let's face it. No one really wants to be responsible for how their life looks, especially if they are sick. Just blame it on something or someone else. It's easier that way. But, *you* are the one responsible for your own life and well-being. It's very easy to get caught up in the blame game and to accept the opinions of these false prophets. They are validating your fear and negative beliefs; as you know, beliefs always seek validation. That's what makes these shows so popular. Many of you have become addicted to experiencing life as a powerless, hapless victim of circumstances beyond your control. That addiction is the result of the ego's resistance. It fears change because it fears annihilation. It takes a leap of faith to let go of your attachment to your conditioning and beliefs, but if you don't, you will remain powerless to create a new model of health and well-being for your life.

When Buddha said that life is suffering, he was no longer identified with ego. He was free from the limitations of ego and conditioning. He said that you suffer because of your attachments. You are unwilling to give up your emotional attachments and addictions because you identify with them.

Robert had the unconscious belief that women always betray him. His ego did not want to release that pattern; as far as it was concerned, that's the way it was for him. Subsequently, I took him through a process that released his emotional attachment to the pattern and cleared it.

If you are miserable, sick, or poor, the ego doesn't really care. It sees its job as maintaining your conditioning and beliefs about reality. Think about this for a moment. You are sick and desperately want to become well, yet you are identified with, and addicted to, the circumstances your ego has accepted as your reality. Your ego would rather see you sick and desperate than to change, because its job is to maintain your reality, no matter *how* painful and debilitating it is. As you begin to understand how your ego works, your resistance to change will diminish. It wants you to be dependent on others for healing. It doesn't want you to know that you have the power to heal yourself, because that's not part of ego's reality. Well-being is your natural state. It's just buried under layers of conditioning and beliefs about how life works.

I'll tell you a story about myself that shows just how diabolical the ego can be. About twenty years ago, I decided it was time to finish healing this lifetime. I had already been in psychotherapy for a long time. I received a lot of benefit from it, but then realized I wasn't getting to my core issues, so stopped going. I didn't know what to do next. Then, one day, while perusing a bookstore about 200 miles from where I lived in Seattle, a place called the tri-cities, in Southeastern Washington State. The names of those towns are Kennewick, Pasco, and Richland. A friend and I were going deer hunting in Eastern Washington. Actually, it was just an excuse to go camping and to drink a little beer in the snow. Passing through Kennewick, we stopped to see if we could find anything to read while we sat by our campfire. As I was looking at the books, one of them practically fell off the shelf into my hands. The title of the book was *The Primal Scream* by Dr. Janhov, a noted psychotherapist. Note the unseen hand of the universe at work here, guiding me to just what I needed at the time, in the same way you have been guided to *this* book.

After reading the book, I decided I wanted to participate in the emotional clearing process described therein, but it would have cost thousands of dollars for me to go to California and work with Dr. Janhov. I just couldn't afford it. A few months later, I was in another bookstore in Edmonds, Washington, about ten miles from where I lived. There were some people putting on what they called a rebirthing session. It seemed to me to be very similar to what Dr. Janhov had described. The demonstration was inexpensive, so I decided to join in. Rebirthing is a process of deep emotional clearing, using the breath. It evoked deep suppressed feelings and emotions just like Dr. Janhov had described in his book. There was a workshop scheduled that would include an entire weekend, so I decided to participate.

Long story short, right after I joined the workshop, I had an automobile accident—actually there *are* no accidents, but that's what I called it at the time. No big deal—my insurance paid to have my car fixed. About a month later, I joined an even longer and more intense workshop.

I had *another* automobile accident. Both of the accidents were my fault. I wasn't hurt badly, just bruised a little, but I nearly crashed into a gasoline tanker. Had that happened, I would have been toast!

My car came close to being totaled and I knew that my insurance would be cancelled. I couldn't shrug this one off. Something very sinister was going on. I went to bed early that evening and woke up in the middle of the night to take some ibuprofen for the pain in my bruised body. Wanting to know why those "accidents" had occurred, I climbed out of bed and sat down in the chair often used for my meditations. With my eyes closed, in a light meditative state, I asked why those accidents had happened. An answer came almost immediately. My inner voice said, "You would rather die than face your fears."

I was stunned. My image was one of seeing myself as a brave and courageous person, but my ego preferred death to facing those unconscious fears.

The next question was, "How do I keep from killing myself?" It said, "Stop driving for two months." I was selling real estate at the time, but I knew if I continued to drive, death was a real possibility. So, even though my insurance company fixed my car, I stopped driving. After about six weeks, I realized the death scenario was cleared. My fears had been faced in the rebirthing workshop and I moved on and started driving again. This is a classic example of how ego despises change and in some cases would rather destroy you than to face change. By hanging onto those fears and old patterns, you believe you are safer and more secure, when in fact, it's just the opposite.

# # #

CHAPTER FIVE
KNOW THYSELF

To know who you are, your strengths, weaknesses, and what motivates your choices, is certainly one of the most challenging things a person can do. Yet, without doing so, life simply becomes a blind acceptance of what you have been led to believe is true. You are driven by motives you don't consciously understand. When asked, most people will tell you they understand themselves quite well, but if you ask them whether they are satisfied with their lives, the answer is no. Of course, everyone has some superficial knowledge of themselves, but the quiet dissatisfaction most people experience speaks of a life in which there is constant inner conflict. Knowing yourself means that you understand yourself emotionally, psychologically, physically, and spiritually.

To understand yourself may seem like a tall order, but it can be easily accomplished if you make the effort and take one step at a time. Self-awareness progresses like a flower opening to the sun. Your Higher Nature and spirituality are the force behind your physical life. It supports what you see in your reflection. Yet, the characteristics of your Higher Nature are very different from what you see in the mirror. Without a better understanding of who you are, you will not find peace or equilibrium. That lack of understanding causes insecurity, stress, and vulnerability to disease.

Chances are you have decided to read this book because you're not having the best of times. In reading this, you may believe you have found a sound plan to restore balance and healing. You may indeed take on the challenge of getting to know and understand yourself. Some people become motivated when their physical maladies fail to respond to traditional medical treatment. Early in the twentieth century, modern medicine established a category of psychosomatic diseases, and then, systematically, discredited or chose to ignore how disease is created. Modern medicine has developed a distorted view of disease.

Medicine ignores the connection of mind to disease, because if they give it any credence, they just might have to explore their *own* emotional makeup; few doctors are willing to do that. The courage to do so speaks highly of your inner strength. Exploring who you are creates change, and as you know, egos deplore change. Individuals often demand change in the outer world, yet are reluctant to make change in their inner world. Let me stress again, the importance of exploring your emotions and feelings. It is a necessary part of the growth and healing process. It takes a disproportional amount of your energy to keep your issues from surfacing. You simply cannot evolve and heal while suppressing your feelings at the same time.

I have worked with many people who displayed tremendous resistance when it came to looking at their feelings and emotions. In all cases, after exploring and clearing those feelings and emotions, they wondered what the big deal had been, and then laughed at their resistance like it was simply a bad joke. As you know, most people prefer changes in their lives to come about because *others* have changed. That's understandable, but it simply isn't the way change occurs.

The belief that others influence your life is an incredible distortion of the way life really works. I have talked about this earlier, but it's worth repeating. Your inner landscape creates your personal experience of your outer world. This externalized view of the world is one perpetuated by societies all over the planet. It ignores the possibility that you alone are responsible for creating the world you experience.

One of Wayne Dyer's popular books from a number of years ago was titled, *You'll See It When You Believe It*. Simply stated, this means that what you see and experience is the result of what you believe about the world you live in. If your inner world is a wonderful, joyous, and abundant place, then that is what you will experience. If you see life as a struggle, filled with disappointment and lack, then that is what you will experience. In even more simple words, Abraham Lincoln is credited as saying, "Most folks are about as happy as they make up their minds to be."

You can find grace in every experience you encounter, even the most negative ones, but you must look for it. Pain is often the most profound teacher. The grace you find will bring a benefit far greater than the illness or negative experiences you have.

Transformation and growth always begin with dissatisfaction. Your life, or some aspect of your life, isn't working, be it financial, a dead-end job, a relationship, or even sickness. When there is great dissatisfaction, suffering, and disappointment in life, you will likely turn inward for answers, because instinctively, you realize there isn't anywhere else to turn. When this happened to me, a series of questions came: "Who am I?" "Why am I here?" "What is my purpose in this lifetime?" These kinds of questions present a great opportunity to discover who you are and to create change. When questions like this start coming to you, it means your Higher Nature has broken through the smoke screen and strategies that your ego has created to avoid change. These are open-ended questions and are not meant to be answered by mind and intellect. The answers will come from within.

"Who am I?" Answering this question goes to the very heart of self-awareness. It is central to your transformation and healing, because it leads you deep into your inner world. The answer will unfold as you evolve. Suffice it to say that you are not your mind, conditioning, beliefs, thoughts, and ego. When all of your ideas about who you are fall away, all that is left is a sense of awareness and truth. That is who you are.

One of the best ways to utilize this question is to ask it as you slip into meditation. Then, just let the answer come to you. Remember, this question doesn't require an answer. It is an open-ended question and answering it with mind will only defeat its purpose. Let me caution you not to rush the process, not to strain for an answer. That will only cause a delay. It could take days, or even weeks, but an answer will come to you, as it did for me. **Answering the question "Who am I?" is the most powerful healing stance you can take.**

Here is an example of how to begin. Pick a quiet, comfortable spot to sit, one in which you can easily relax. Go into a light, meditative state or simply relax. Close your eyes and ask yourself, "Who am I?" Repeat the question several times. Then, let go, surrender, and notice what's there before you start thinking again. You don't have to devote a lot of time to this, a few minutes each day is enough. It's not easy to describe who you are, but you will know it when you experience it. Most likely it will come to you as a "feeling," or you may experience a vast "emptiness." Just notice what is there when your thoughts stop. For some of you, your mind is so active that your thoughts rarely stop. That's the way it was for me when I began this adventure. Now, I can slip into that timeless, thoughtless state almost any time and it only takes a moment or two.

This is a shortcut to discovering who you are. It is referred to as self-inquiry, in some of the Eastern teachings. Some of you will be drawn to this process, others will not. If it seems just a little too vague or obscure after trying it a few times, that's OK. You can come back to it later. I admit that the process of self-inquiry just wasn't for me when I began my own healing and transformation. This is actually a process of reintegration with your Higher Nature.

While there may be a number of reasons you are here, the primary one is to experience who you are *not*. You are here to explore the limitations of being physical and what it's like to be totally involved in duality and the relative world of opposites. You have come to play the "limitation game" and now that you have experienced it ad nauseam, you are ready to resume your authority over your life. Chapter Ten talks about purpose.

A little about duality and the nature of the world you live in: one of the major problems you face throughout life is the dualistic nature of the world you live in; duality means opposites. With duality there is a tendency for everything to turn to its opposite—here today, gone tomorrow. You see this in so many areas of life, even in the political systems. This is the reason political solutions are so difficult. You may have a wonderful solution to a problem, yet no matter how good it is, someone will oppose it.

This disintegration is the nature of the world you live in. It is hard-wired into your brain. It's part of your neural network. You may have noticed the tendency for opposition within yourself and in your relationships. It's one of the reasons relationships are so difficult to maintain. You may be wondering how this can ever be changed, and how we can truly develop an open mind and be receptive to new ideas and to others. You will find as you grow and evolve, this tendency for opposition will begin to diminish. It is the identification with conditioning and ego that sustains duality. As you experience more of who you are, you will become more integrated with your Higher Nature. All personal growth and healing are the result of becoming more integrated and balanced.

One of the reasons you have become so disintegrated is because of the tendency to make things complex. This tendency is the result of relying on science and analysis to solve problems, instead of relying on your inner wisdom, intuition, and heart. Medical science always wants to complicate the healing process. You may think science is a way of discovering truth, but as I said earlier, science is simply just another belief system.

You never actually lose your connection with your Higher Nature. You just lose sight of it and are not aware of it. That's why integration is possible and comparatively simple. A few minutes each day is all it takes. Another aspect of the dualistic world is right and wrong. Of course, right and wrong are purely subjective opinions. There is no absolute right or wrong, yet it looks that way. Those who blew up the twin towers in New York City and killed almost 3,000 people were convinced that they were right and God was on *their* side.

When you give up the idea of right and wrong, you will begin to experience more integration with your Higher Nature. Maybe you think that if we were to give up the idea of right and wrong, there would be more destruction and chaos in the world, yet, the way things are playing out, we are destroying the world *anyway*.

In his book, *The Tao of Physics,* Fritjof Capra has this to say about the way duality is created: "Opposites are abstract concepts belonging to the realm of thought, and as such, they are relative. By the very act of focusing our attention on any one concept, we create its opposite. As Lao

Tzu says: 'When all in the world understand beauty to be beautiful, then ugliness exists; when all understand goodness to be good, then evil exists.' Mystics transcend this realm of intellectual concepts, and in transcending it, become aware of the relativity and polar relationship of all opposites. They realize that good and bad, pleasure and pain, life and death, are not absolute experiences belonging to different categories, but are merely two sides of the same reality extreme parts of a single whole. The awareness that all opposites are polar and thus a unity, is seen as one of the highest aims of man in the spiritual traditions of the East. 'Be in truth eternal, beyond earthly opposite' is Krishna's advice in the Bhagavad-Gita, and the same advice is given to the followers of Buddhism."

Much of what you see as right and wrong is the result of ego's need to be right. Ego's sense of power comes from seeing itself as right and others as wrong. Out of right and wrong comes ego's need for conflict.

Everyone I've worked with has what I call unconscious contracts or agreements that they have made with family members. In many families, they will share a certain disease. It looks like its hereditary, but actually, it is the result of conditioning and subtle, unconscious programming. It may even have begun in the womb: to not be more successful than your parents (or other family members), or to carry on family traditions passed down from generation to generation, such as sexual or physical abuse, and poverty. Your family heritage goes back generations and can be passed down to you genetically. Your ancestors have invested a great deal of energy in them. Those contracts are deeply unconscious and rarely questioned. You may be totally unaware of your agreement to fulfill those behavioral patterns, but you will pass them on to the next generation, just as your parents did. After all, the family cherishes its traditions, even the negative ones. Only those who are willing to explore the depths of their own contracts will break the chains that keep them from being passed on to the next generation. Your family will not like you exposing their secrets, but it is the only way you can stop living out their dysfunctional behaviors.

Mary had a degree in architecture. She was the most educated person in her family, the only one to attend college. She was employed by various companies and any time that she was up for a promotion, something would get in the way. Often, it was a medical problem that kept her away from work for long periods, sometimes for several months. By the time she came to see me, she was already looking for work in a different field.

The dissatisfaction she felt around her career was blamed on the type of work she had chosen to do. But, like so many other people, she had decided that outside forces beyond her control were interfering with her life. As we explored her inner world, we found that she had subconsciously formed contracts with members of her family that she would not exceed *their* accomplishments. For her, the strongest agreement was with her older sister. This was her way of placating an older sister when she was very young, but it had carried over into adulthood, as contracts made by children so often do. Once she became aware of the problem, she was able to overcome it and get on with her life.

The most difficult exploration usually occurs when you explore your feelings and emotions. In this culture, both men and women have been taught that expressing emotions is somehow bad, or harmful. Clinical studies show that there is great relief from tension and anxiety by surrendering to the simple act of crying. Anyone who has explored emotional release can attest to the catharsis that occurs when deeply suppressed emotions surface and are experienced.

As I have traveled the planet, worked with, taught, and participated with both small and large groups of people, it has become clear to me that the majority of people who live in the Western world are suppressing their emotions and feelings.

As you grow, you will begin to give up your personal will. If you are strong-willed and ego-centered, you are most likely affronted by the thought of giving up your personal will. Almost everyone believes that their success is dependent on their own personal strength, will, and even their power of persuasion. Your success in this world is much more dependent upon your personal connection to your Higher Nature than from any qualities of the personality. Wisdom, intuition, and creativity are far more critical to your ultimate success. These can easily be blocked by your emotions and personal will. Many people will try to avoid giving up personal will, but everyone has to grow up at some time, look at their issues, and stop blaming the outer world for their plight.

Self-awareness does not come cheap. It requires an investment of energy and a dedication to knowing thyself. This is the real work of those who truly want to grow and heal, as well as those who wish to attain true success.

Sometimes great inspiration comes as the result of the simple act of contemplation or meditation. Many of my ideas come while bicycling or walking. The inspiration for this book came to me while waking up one morning. It isn't possible to begin to know yourself without first turning inward. Of course, there is always the chance that you will find deeply buried emotions, memories, even traumatic events that you would rather not look at, but you are just as likely to find marvelous, wonderful qualities, and aspects of yourself that you did not even know were there. It certainly never occurred to me that I could become a writer until I began to explore my inner nature. I find the act of writing to be a wonderful, creative experience, one that lay completely dormant until I began to go inward. The deeper meaning for your own life may very well be suppressed beneath your feelings. Without being able to feel, you become numb to life, suffer, and struggle.

Your lifetime on this emerald green planet is a Divine plan. You arrived here, equipped with the skills, abilities, aptitudes, and whatever else it takes to survive, heal, and experience the joy of life. What seems to plague many individuals is a sense that they are hopelessly flawed. These thoughts are just another clever ruse of ego, designed to keep you focused on your limitations. Ego gets its sense of identity from the past. No matter how small a change may be, it sees it as a threat to its very existence.

As you go inward, you'll begin to take on qualities of your Higher Nature; perhaps fleetingly at first, but nevertheless, those qualities will begin to emerge. You may never have thought of uncovering your own spiritual nature, but in fact, it is there. Like so many other undiscovered parts of yourself, it is simply buried under a lot of debris. Many, who have discovered great, latent qualities and gifts, are digging even deeper to see what else is there.

Joy and happiness come from experiencing your soul's uniqueness. Self-awareness unlocks the gifts of your soul and its connection to the universe. You will uncover your real strength, creativity, and ability to heal. You will come to know yourself and be able to perfect the art of self-awareness. Knowing yourself is simply a metaphor for creating self-awareness and connection with your Higher Nature. The little selves you find along the way are really only relative selves. They have been conditioned and trained in this artificial reality, creating limitations and even disease. Those selves will be transient and will hang around for awhile until you release them one at a time. This gives you the opportunity to move forward and explore the *next* layer.

You may notice some repetition as you read along, but it is purposeful and necessary. The repetition will begin to change your belief about how your life and disease are created, and it will accelerate your healing.

# # #

CHAPTER SIX
HEALING AND BELIEF

In difficult times, you absolutely must maintain a positive, can-do attitude. When you allow yourself to become demoralized, your energy contracts and you are not receptive to healing. It's the old adage, "Your attitude affects your altitude." Maintaining a positive attitude may be difficult when times are tough, but it is important to turning your health and fortune around. Actually, what you have to do is stop negative thinking, because it lowers your frequencies. As you know, energy follows thought. Doubt is the culprit. It triggers negative emotions and starts a downward spiral that leads to hopelessness and despair. From there, you will find it difficult to heal and turn your life around. What is actually happening is your heart center is contracting and you will not be able to receive healing, or love.

You don't have to ignore the facts and go into denial, but it does mean you have to stay detached and not follow the crowd into a burning building. As I am writing this, thousands of people are being diagnosed with cancer. You cannot avoid hearing a lot of dire news and commentary. So, monitor your thoughts and don't allow yourself to get caught up in the hysteria. One way to maintain a positive attitude is to read inspirational articles, stories, and books where people have miraculously survived cancer and other life-threatening diseases.

There is a universal law at work here, The Law of Abundance. It is usually talked about when discussing financial matters and acquiring things, but it applies to health and well-being, as well. This law is governed by acceptance. It says, "You receive that which you are able to accept." The universe is on your side. It is always sending you gifts and well-being, but you may not be able to accept them, because of those negative patterns in your unconscious mind. Stop! Think about this. You desire to heal, but you have beliefs in your unconscious mind that oppose what you want. It goes without saying, that if you are not able to accept what the universe is sending, you will never get it. Again, the inability to accept what you desire comes from beliefs in your unconscious mind.

Express appreciation and gratitude for the support you receive from family and friends. The love they have for you is important and assists you with healing. Appreciation opens your heart center and makes you more receptive to health and well-being. One of the keys to healing lies in your willingness to accept love. It is very likely that if you are experiencing poor health, you are also having difficulty accepting love. Often, the belief keeping you from love is the same one that creates sickness. Many of you have a belief that you don't deserve love. If you cannot let love in, then health and well-being will elude you. Love is the healing force. Fear creates limitation and disease.

There is another universal law that is critical to your health, The Law of Mind. It says, "As you believe, so shall you receive." The Bible says, "It is done unto you according to your belief." Everything you experience is subject to this law. There are no exceptions. The Law of Mind cannot be violated. The Law of Mind can be a great benefactor or a terrible task master.

Most doctors and healers are unaware of The Law of Mind. As a result, they lead their clients to believe they can create well-being without doing something about their negative beliefs. Once a belief is created, it will dominate your experience from that point on, or until it is cleared.

Some believe that positive thinking is the key to achieving good health. Thought can play a part in health, but often it's a negative one. The mind cannot process a negative. When you say to yourself, "I don't want to be sick," the mind recognizes only the word sick and activates it. That soon becomes exactly what you are creating, so watch your thoughts, self-talk, and the stories you tell yourself. No single thought will create a belief, but many similar thoughts over a period of time, will create a belief. Often, beliefs are created by the way you feel about something.

You are autonomous. It doesn't matter what's going on around you, there is nothing outside of you that can affect you. Quantum physics says, the "observer" creates the "observed." You are the observer and creator of your life and no one, or no thing, has any power over you.

You exist in a hologram; you are self-contained. Nothing lies outside of it. Everything you want to create already exists within your hologram, including good health. The following is an excerpt from the book *Busting Loose from the Money Game,* by Robert Scheinfield: "Many scientists on the cutting edge of quantum physics and related research believe the hologram is the perfect metaphor to illustrate how the physical universe is made.

"If you saw the movie, 'The Matrix,' or you've seen a 'Star Trek' movie or television show where the characters used the 'holodeck,' you've seen what's really possible with holograms."

Here is the best description I've found of what a hologram is and how it is created. It is from Dr. Stephen

Wolinsky's book, *Quantum Consciousness:* "A hologram is a three-dimensional photograph manufactured with the aid of a laser. To make a hologram, scientists first shine a laser beam on an object, and then, bounce a second laser beam off the reflected light of the first. Interestingly, it is the pattern of interference created by the two lasers that is recorded on a piece of film to create a hologram. To the naked eye, the image recorded on such a piece of film is a meaningless swirl. However, if another laser beam is shown through the developed film, the image reappears in all of its original and three-dimensional glory.

"In addition to being three-dimensional, the image recorded in a hologram differs from a conventional photograph in another very important way. If you cut a normal photograph in half, each section will contain only half of the image that was contained in the original photograph. This is because each tiny section of the photograph, like each dot on a color television, contains only a single bit of information about the entire image.

"However, if you cut a hologram in half and then shine a laser through one of the sections, you will find that each half still contains the entire image of the original hologram. Each tiny section of the hologram contains not only its own bit of information, but every other bit of information from the rest of the image as well. Thus, you can cut a hologram up into pieces and each individual piece will still contain a blurred, but complete version of the entire picture. In other words, in a hologram, every part of the image inter-penetrates every other part in the same way that Bohm's non-local universe would inter-penetrate all of its parts."

There are millions of forms or templates in your hologram and unconscious mind; however, they are dormant until energized. Once a template is energized, it becomes a belief. Working in concert with your Higher Nature, you can decide how your life will look. You can turn off an old, outdated pattern and replace it with a new one. Your Higher Nature uses mind to energize what it wants to create. Once it becomes an energized pattern or a belief, thought takes over and gives it direction, like a bullet traveling toward a target. Almost all teachers and healers tell you to focus on what you are trying to create, but when you do that, you are putting your energy into the result, instead of the point of creation. It's like starting a race at the finish line. Instead, put your focus on your Higher Nature; it is the healing force.

Here is a simple technique for connecting with your Higher Nature. Do this whenever you are feeling stress or simply need more clarity and direction. It is a way of focusing on your essence and Higher Nature. Notice it's the same technique used when doing Vipassana meditation, but is abbreviated. Just close your eyes, breathe deeply, relax, and put all of your attention on your breathing. Breathe a little deeper than you would ordinarily. Follow your breath in and out for a minute or two. At the end of the process, simply notice what's there before you start thinking again. Another benefit of this technique is that it will connect you to your wisdom self, for answers or solutions to problems. The information you are looking for may come right away, or it may take two to three minutes.

Here is another simple technique to help you strengthen your connection to your Higher Nature: Sit down, close your eyes, and put yourself in a light meditative state. Create a symbol for your Higher Nature. It can be any symbol, the sun, the moon, or even your favorite teddy bear—whatever feels right for you. I use the Milky Way Galaxy as a symbol for *my* Higher Nature. Suspend your thoughts and intensely focus on the symbol you have chosen. It is just that simple. Do this daily and it will strengthen your connection.

It is either "obstacle" or "flow." Obstacles are negative feelings and thoughts that have solidified into a belief. Healing is there for you on the other side of those obstacles. In order to clear negative beliefs, you need to first find and identify them. Here are two approaches you can take at this point. You can make a list of limiting beliefs from what you experience, or you can use the emotional discomfort you feel to identify what needs to be cleared. I do both. Sometimes I make a list and write them down, or I explore the discomfort that I feel. If you choose to write them down, take a look at your life and ask yourself, what issues do I currently experience? You can call on your Higher Nature to help you find those obstacles. It will do so with great enthusiasm and effectiveness.

Often, there will be a cluster of patterns around a particular belief. A belief such as, "I am always sick," will be supported by beliefs around not deserving to be healthy: "I don't deserve to be strong and healthy." "I don't deserve to feel good." Others on your list may include: "I don't deserve to get what I want" or "I never get what I want." "I am powerless to change." "Nothing ever works out." "My efforts never pay off." "I am undeserving." "I'm not valued." "No one values my efforts." "I am unworthy." "I don't deserve love." You will find many others and your list will expand.

Open your eyes and take a good look at what you are experiencing. Your life is reflecting back to you what you believe. No exceptions. If you don't like what you see, you have the power to create change, but your ego wants you to believe that you don't. You will find it very difficult to heal your life, if at the same time you are replicating those old patterns and beliefs.

Love is the primary healing force. If you are feeling unloved, it is because you don't believe you are worthy or deserve love. Or, that God has abandoned you. God cannot, and will not, abandon you, even though you may believe that he has. You will not be abandoned, even if you are an atheist. God didn't create the universe; He *became* the universe, so whether you know it or not, *you* are your Higher Nature. It is always with you.

We have a special word for those who challenge your beliefs; they are called heretics and the penalty for being a heretic can be very harsh. During much of our planet's history, the penalty was death for those who threatened our beliefs. Now, all that happens is that you will be castigated, shunned, scorned, or ridiculed. That's all.

As a child, you had to go along with familial and cultural beliefs or you would be punished or perhaps even killed. A child certainly can't afford to be shunned by its family and peers.

Here is the process for clearing beliefs. You have written down a belief or have discovered an uncomfortable feeling and have identified it as something you want to clear. Maybe you feel discomfort while shopping for groceries and feel like you can't clear it while standing in the checkout line. I have actually cleared patterns while waiting in line at the grocery store. If you are not comfortable doing this, then after you return home, sit down and ask your Higher Nature to show you the feeling and discomfort you experienced while shopping. Just close your eyes, take a deep breath, and go into a light meditative state, or simply close your eyes, relax, and ask your Higher Nature to show you what needs to be cleared.

It doesn't matter if you can actually find the belief or emotional pattern. You can create a symbol for it with your imagination and *pretend* to find it. That works just as well as actually finding it. Your intention to find it will take you to the pattern, whether you are aware of it or not. Be sure to allow yourself to breathe deeply. Holding your breath is how this pattern got suppressed in the first place.

Next, dive into the pattern and feel it as deeply as you can. Stay with the feeling and immerse yourself in the energy of the pattern. It may begin to intensify. Stay with the intensity as best you can. You will never get more than you can handle. When you feel like the intensity has peaked, ask your Higher Nature to transmute it or release the energy from the belief. Initially, you may not be aware of what is going on, but like any other skill, it will improve with practice. To make it more noticeable, ask your Higher Nature to strengthen your experience.

Your attitude has to be—bring it on! Stand your ground. Don't wimp out on yourself. Your ego will try to distract you from this work, if it can. The quality of your life is at stake here. It takes courage to change.

Devote twenty minutes daily, or every other day, to the process. If you commute by bus or train, you can do the clearing at that time. Typically, when I begin clearing, I start yawning like crazy. It's the way I release energy. If that happens to you, it might be a little distracting to the person sitting next to you, but so what? Do it anyway. It's your life!

There have been times when I sat down for only five minutes to clear a pattern and other times when I have spent an hour or more clearing a number of patterns. Exactly what works best for you will unfold. And, remember, in some strange way, your ego is smarter than you are. It will try to divert and distract you from the process. One client of mine got dizzy and confused and her mind fogged over when she started clearing. That was her ego's resistance. Talk to your ego; ask it to step aside and to support what is best for you. It will relent if you just stand your ground. You will probably find that you'll have to go over your list many times before those old patterns will be totally cleared.

How do you know when you are making progress? You will begin healing and your life will start to change. Be patient. It will happen for you just like it has for me and for many others. If you have not yet learned to go inward, and have little self-awareness, it may take longer. I am talking about creating a new paradigm. Your intention and commitment to do this work is the most important ally you possess—along with your bring-it-on attitude!

Let's say you have been clearing patterns for several months and you are not responding as quickly as you would like to; something keeps reoccurring in your life that isn't to your liking. You keep looking for the pattern, but no matter how hard you try, it won't raise its ugly head so you can cut it off.

Resistance is the problem. Your ego is saying, "No way!" Do not directly confront your ego's resistance. Don't challenge it. If you do, it will simply become stronger. You can clear your resistance the same way you clear any other pattern. Just dive into it, acknowledge it, and ask your Higher Nature to transmute it or let the energy out of it. Some beliefs are tenacious and difficult to clear. As you clear the patterns around it that help keep it in place, it will begin to surface so you can clear it. How long will it take to see a change? You will probably see some change right away, but it can take longer in some cases, even a month or more.

While exploring old, repressed beliefs, you may find that emotions, memories, and intense feelings come to the surface. This is a good news/bad news scenario. The bad news is that it's uncomfortable. The good news is the patterns are coming up to be cleared. Your Higher Nature is creating this response; it knows exactly what it is doing. Remember, you will never get more than you can handle.

Suppressed feelings that are not cleared will eventually create physical symptoms and disease. Some people would rather have the physical pain than the emotional discomfort. It's your choice. However, the physical pain is always much more severe. The process for clearing emotions and feelings is the same one used for clearing beliefs.

When working with clients, it usually takes three or four sessions before they begin to go deeply within and start clearing in earnest. Give yourself the necessary time. You have been suppressing your feelings since you were an infant.

According to Norman Cousins, the author of *The Anatomy of an Illness,* "Drugs are not always necessary. Belief in recovery always is." If you allow your ego to divert your attention from the process, your life will not change and you will continue to experience illness. You can choose to be courageous, or you can give up on yourself.

You can approach this process as though it is punishment perpetrated by a demanding, cruel universe (at times, it may be somewhat unpleasant), or you can accept it as a gift from the universe to heal and free you from bondage.

As you know by now, all disease is the result of suppressed feelings, emotion, beliefs, and thought forms in your unconscious mind. You must release those old, suppressed patterns in order to heal. It's up to *you* to explore those feelings and patterns; no one can do it for you, however, there is universal support available to you.

As you heal and evolve, you will reintegrate with your Higher Nature. Perhaps you have little or no interest in personal evolution and reintegration with your Higher Nature. That's okay. It's perfectly fine. But you may not heal as quickly. **Within every illness there is a gift, an opportunity for growth, healing, and renewal.**

You may think this process is too simple to be effective. Modern medicine has invested billions of dollars in complicated technologies and it wants you to think that complexity is a necessary part of healing, but it isn't.

Healing occurs because it is a natural phenomenon; it has nothing to do with complexity. The only thing standing between you and your well-being are those old thought forms, emotions, and feelings that are buried in your unconscious mind. They can easily be cleared.

# # #

CHAPTER SEVEN
THE NATURAL FLOW OF LIFE

Theoretically, living in the twenty-first century with all of the technology and modern conveniences you enjoy, life should be easier for everyone. Still, for many, there is a gradual erosion of the quality of their lives. No doubt you have a sense that something is changing the very fabric of the world you live in. This perception is accurate. What you are experiencing is an energy shift. The energies that have supported the cultural and medical systems of the world in the past are evolving and changing. A new paradigm is being created for humanity. You have been trained to work and compete in an era where conditions were very different from what they are today. You were taught to live and work within a paradigm that is no longer valid. The truth is that the old ways never really worked, it only seemed that way. Life may seem chaotic and uncertain, but it's always that way when a new paradigm is being birthed.

You grew up in a male-dominated, patriarchal society in which the theme was "control." A patriarchal system is a take-charge, rigid, and unimaginative system in which whoever can fight their way to the top is the king of the hill. Leaders are worshipped and respected, simply because they are in authority. Make no mistake, the paradigm your grandparents and their grandparents operated from will not work for you in your life today. Of course, it did not really work for them either. You can see the old guard continually trying to re-establish itself. When things go wrong, how do those in charge respond? They establish more laws and regulations. This piling on of controls is what has brought our society to its current state of dysfunction, trapped behind the doors to your homes, if you are fortunate enough to *have* a home. Individually, and as a whole, you are losing ground fast. Control does not work. In order to make your life work, you must stop trying to control it. Your ego loves control. It gives it a sense of power.

I was raised in a family where iron-fisted will and physical courage were all that mattered. You got what you wanted out of life by force of will, with a little manipulation added, in case force alone was not enough. In my mid-twenties, I went into business for myself. For a number of years, I was successful at applying what I had learned as a child, which was the exact opposite of the meek inheriting the earth. In our household, the meek were stepped on or pushed out of the way. After a number of years in business, things gradually began to go wrong. My response was to apply more control and more force of will. In the past, this was always a solution, but I found that after a certain point, force of will no longer worked. My therapist at the time suggested that I give up control, sit back and listen to what was being said by my employees, and then to allow *them* to take charge. So, that is exactly what I did. Immediately, my business began to right itself and return to profit. This was my first experience of consciously giving up control, but certainly not my last. To this day, I find that surrendering and staying out of control takes constant vigilance. It is by no means easy to give up your childhood conditioning. Controllers are often angry people. Control contracts your energies and distorts them.

The universe is a loving, supporting place in which you are never alone. There is a Divine intelligence; call it your Higher Nature, or God if you choose, which guides the planet through its orbit around the sun, creating the seasons, day, and night. It beats your heart and spins the atoms that make up your body; it provides the divine spark for your existence. Be assured that there is a plan for your life that was conceived by that intelligence. This blueprint, when followed, will bring you true fulfillment and satisfaction.

When disease strikes, it is because you are in conflict with the natural order and flow of your life. The simple truth is that there is a natural order and flow to life that affects everything. All of your successes in life, whether large or small, are the result of your alignment with the natural order of the universe. People have sought to live outside of the natural flow, in a kind of no-man's land. When you are connected with your Higher Nature and not judging the events of your life as good or bad, life will flow effortlessly.

So, exactly who is in charge of your life? Your ego? Your soul? Your Higher Nature? The truth is that there is a natural process of co-creation between you and your Higher Nature, that is, when you are not attempting to create by edict and force of will. Living from flow is exactly the opposite of taking charge of your life. Up until this point, you have been trying in vain to take charge. It is time for you to surrender the grip you hold on your reality, and allow the natural process of co-creation and healing to proceed.

Ego is pleasure seeking, and will avoid pain at all costs. Pain and suffering may seem like a natural part of your life, but they are the result of resistance and control. Loss of a job or the break-up of a relationship are perceived by most as very painful. Yet, death is part of life. An end to things as you know them simply opens the door for something better in the future. When you yield and accept what is going on in your life, you begin to restore peace and equilibrium.

Some people believe you have just one lifetime in which to get it right, but that belief is very limited and untrue. You may be uncertain about this concept, but I am convinced that we have many lifetimes, because I remember some of them, especially the last one.

One Saturday morning a number of years ago, I decided to take a trip to McMinnville, Oregon, where a friend of mine was putting on a channeling event in a local bookstore. This was something new to me at that time, and I was curious about it. McMinnville is about two hundred miles south of Seattle, where I lived at the time, and forty miles southwest of Portland, Oregon.

McMinnville was a sleepy little town that had been built at the turn-of-the-twentieth century. Life centered around a main street consisting of hotels, boarding houses, and other businesses. Historically, McMinnville was founded by William T. Newby, who had traveled to Oregon from McMinnville, Tennessee, on the first wagon train during the Great Migration of 1843. The town was established by 1882, with a building boom occurring around the turn-of-the-twentieth century. Many of the original buildings are still intact.

The area around McMinnville is dotted with picturesque vineyards and colorful fields of blooming clover during the summertime. Another point of interest is the Evergreen Aviation Museum, housing the Spruce Goose, the world's largest propeller-driven airplane. It was designed and built by the famous aviator and eccentric billionaire, Howard Hughes. Constructed completely from wood, due to wartime raw material shortages, it made its only flight in 1947.

After I arrived in town, I decided to take a stroll down the main street. As I walked past an old, turn-of-the century building with retail businesses on the street level and apartments on the second floor, I glanced up a stairway leading to the second floor. I had an immediate reaction. The energy emanating from the building caused me to feel strange and uneasy. I felt like I was in the right place, but at the wrong time. Suddenly, I became aware that I had been propelled back in time to when I had worked as a building contractor in McMinnville. In the early 1900s, my name at the time was John and I had migrated to McMinnville from Montana in the early 1900s, to become involved in the West Coast building boom. I was a big man; stoop shouldered, drank too much, and was a philanderer. As I walked on, I continued to feel disoriented and uncomfortable. I returned to the book store a little later to observe what was going on, but the feeling of timelessness stayed with me. Later that night, I had dinner with my friend and talked about what I had experienced. She conveyed that she had had a similar experience.

As I drove out of town the next morning, I noticed a large, old house that was about to be torn down. I remembered living in it. Reflecting back on the experience, I realize I was experiencing a "time warp." It was like having one foot in the present and the other in the past. I have not been back to McMinnville since that time, but I intend to return sometime in the future to see if I can acquire more information about that lifetime. According to quantum physics, time does not actually exist. Time is hard-wired into our brain so that we can experience it, but it's really just an illusion.

All of the major religions—Buddhism, Christianity, Hinduism, and the Muslim religion, have spoken of reincarnation. The Bible talked about it until it was taken out by the church at the Second Council of Constantinople in 553 A.D. The reason the church purged it was because they wanted people to focus on the here and now, and not be distracted by the possibility of redemption in another lifetime. This of course, gave the priests more control over their subjects.

Acceptance is paramount; accepting your experience takes you out of control and puts you into the flow of life. Look for the gift of grace in everything that happens, no matter how dire. You will always find the gift when you look for it. No matter how negative you view the experience, there is always something far greater to learn and understand.

The intelligence of the Divine mind which created you resides in your personal energies, and even in the cells of your body. The intelligence of the universe is accessible only when you are centered and in the moment. Maybe you don't believe there is a Divine plan for your life. Life is just a crapshoot. Man, in his arrogance, thinks he is creating a better life for his children by taking charge of his destiny, but the ignorance and chaos seen everywhere certainly speaks of something else.

When you elect new leaders in this democracy (who rarely ever lead), you choose those whom you think can gain control over whatever seems to be out of control; the economy, drugs, and violence in the streets. However, real change is always the result of growth. Of course, the more out of control things get, the harder society and individuals try to grasp the reigns.

Like most people, I've been exposed to the idea of karma for many years and have wondered what it actually is. It has become part of the lexicon of our language. Actually, I've heard talk show hosts and news anchors use it on their programs. What they were implying is that karma is "payback" for wrong doing, but it is much more than that. Of course, *they* are the official arbitrators of right and wrong. I talked earlier about the concept of right and wrong and how, although it is accepted theory, it's dubious at best.

Does karma play a role in your life, or is it just a myth? The answer is that karma plays an important role. It is discussed in the ancient Vedic texts, Buddhism, and many other spiritual and religious teachings. Even the Bible tells us you reap what you sow. This is a reference to the way karma works. The ancient Vedic texts were written when there was very little karma on the planet. As a result, they are not distorted. Exactly when The Vedas were written remains a mystery, but they pre-date any of the ancient cultures that have left a historical record. Of course, you can only have karma when you have duality—when things can be out of balance and lack integration.

In the mid-1990s, I spent time in Thailand. I traveled there to study and meditate with a Vedic scholar. There were about forty of us who went to meditate and study the ancient traditions and knowledge. We stayed at The Royal Ping Resort, located about twenty miles north of Chiang Mai, Thailand's second largest city. The resort is very remote and quiet, and not far from the Burmese border. The resort used to be the summer home for the king and queen of Thailand. It's now a tourist attraction and a place to go for a weekend getaway. It sits on about forty acres of landscaped gardens, next to the meandering Ping River. It is very picturesque and is surrounded by lush forests. One of the unique qualities is that all of the tourist cabins are made out of teak planks, harvested from the nearby forests. There is a Thai village across the way with about fifty inhabitants. Behind the resort, lives a hill tribe of native, indigenous people who have not changed their way of life for centuries. Neither village is visible from the resort. Every morning, at dawn, chickens from the hill tribe came down to the resort, looking for delicious bugs to eat, and the roosters started crowing. I must say, it was a little distracting to my early morning meditation!

On the grounds, there is a large outdoor restaurant with unbelievably delicious Thai food. It is an ideal place for a meditation retreat. There is lots of hustle and bustle in its two major cities, Chiang Mai and Bangkok. Other than that, it's an idyllic place—slow paced, quiet, and serene.

The religion of Thailand is Buddhism and everyone there understands how karma affects us. There are many temples throughout the countryside, and some of them are hundreds, even thousands of years old. The energy of the temples is captivating. In one of the temples I visited, a monk had died many years before; his body was still on display and showed no signs of decomposing. There is a two-thousand-year old temple not far from Chiang Mai that has a bone fragment on display from the remains of Buddha.

Often, you will hear the melodic chanting of the monks, coming from the temples. They are incredibly beautiful and enchanting places to meditate and worship. The temples are imbued with hundreds, even thousands of years of energy produced by chanting and other Buddhist ceremonies.

After a few days of meditating nearly around the clock, I slipped into a state of timelessness. The only breaks we had from meditation were meals and ten minutes of yoga exercises every two or three hours, plus an afternoon lecture on The Vedas. The reason for the yoga exercises was to move the karma that got stirred up during meditation. Meditation is a very effective way to release karma.

Even though I was in a timeless state during meditation, there were times when I was very aware of the outside world, and often, time would slow dramatically. Bob Fickes, the teacher and facilitator of the workshop, explained that when time slowed dramatically, we were moving large blocks of karma. Once it was cleared, we would slip back into timelessness. Even though I was there meditating for a month, it seemed like only a few days.

Coming back into a world dominated by time can be very difficult and it can take days to readjust.

While in meditation, I asked to see what karma actually looks like. What was presented to me looked like flies caught on fly paper. The tiny, dark specs represented karma. Fly paper may not exist any more; I don't recall seeing any since I was a child. For those of you who have not seen fly paper, it is a roll of coiled paper, about one-inch wide, suspended from the ceiling and coated with a sticky substance that traps flies. There was a lot of fly paper around in the 1940s and 1950s when I was a child, especially on the farm in North Dakota where I spent my summers. The farm was owned by my aunt and uncle. There was fly paper everywhere you looked; it must have been very inexpensive. Of course there were no pressurized cans of insect spray at that time. It didn't seem all that effective to me, but I guess it made them feel better, more in control, and on the offensive with those pesky critters.

Karma is the driving force behind what you experience in this lifetime. Your conditioning is the result of your karma. For instance, you may have chosen an abusive family so you would have the opportunity to heal and transcend your karma and abuse.

Your conditioning becomes the content of your mind and is filled with false assumptions about the nature of reality. Nearly everyone believes what they learned as a child is true, but it is nearly 100 percent false. Not long ago, I sensed I needed to clear some obstacles in my energy field. I sat back, closed my eyes, went into a light meditative state and was shown what I needed to clear. I didn't actually *see* the karma this time—instead, I felt and sensed it. What I did then was to ask my Higher Nature to do the clearing for me.

In Sanskrit, the word karma means "incomplete action." As you know, the universe is self-correcting and it placed you into this lifetime where you can become aware of the need to heal and clear your karma. Disease is a result of your karma and conditioning. It's up to you whether you to heal, or not. Sooner or later, in one lifetime or another, you *will* choose to heal and balance your karma.

While in Thailand, I went to a sala, a place where the local villagers congregate for healing. Western medicine is available in Thailand for a mere ten percent of the cost of medicine here in the U.S., but it's still too expensive for many of the villagers.

The word sala means "place of healing." The process used is called Thai shamanic healing. It is a Buddhist practice and has been handed down through the centuries, to the villagers; it is directed by Buddha. Petri lives on-site and she is the one in charge. She channels Buddha and has done so for more than forty years. Until I witnessed Petri channeling, I thought it was purely a Western phenomenon. She is perhaps the most skillful channeler I have heard.

Thai shamanic healing uses five elements: air, fire, water, earth, and ether, to facilitate healing. Ether is the space you exist in. There is a very strong emphasis on releasing karma. It's all energy work in one form or another. All of the work is done outside. The main healing area is covered, but there are no walls. Thailand has a tropical climate; it's always warm, sometimes even downright hot, and it rains frequently.

A person must work as an apprentice for many years at the sala in order to become a practitioner. After finishing the apprenticeship, you are initiated into the fraternity of shamans. The personal work and training builds a substantial power base for the individual, and the initiation promotes additional power.

One of the primary tools used to deliver energy is smoke. It is transmitted by a man or woman smoking a cigar. It is no ordinary cigar. They are made of 108 herbs and a small amount of organic tobacco. As the facilitator blows smoke into your nose, a small amount of it is inhaled. After a few seconds it is exhaled. It sounds a little gross, but most people are able to take in smoke rather easily. Within a few seconds of exhaling the smoke, there is an explosion of energy throughout the body and a massive amount of karma is released. The cigars are rolled by a little old lady who lives at the sala. Many diseases are routinely healed in this way. Petri has become so powerful that just a little smoke from her can make it impossible to stand.

The practitioners at the sala are very aware of spirit possession and routinely deal with it when people come for healing. One such experience occurred with one of the members of our group. A friend and fellow meditator was sitting next to me at one of the healing events. One of the practitioners walked directly toward us when suddenly he sprayed water on her, from his mouth. My friend immediately began writhing on the floor, and soon a number of facilitators came to support her. A spirit was being released from her field. It was very similar to the exorcism portrayed in the movie, *The Exorcist.* The spirit was that of a cousin of hers who had been brutally stabbed to death ten years earlier; it had been with her ever since. Mary said that even though the "release" was very dramatic, she hardly knew what was going on. The water sprayed from the practitioner's mouth is called mantra water. It is made each morning by a number of practitioners blowing energy through straws, into a container filled with water. At the same time, others are chanting over it. The water becomes infused with healing energy.

No one wants to be in opposition to universal principles, but you have learned this behavior from your parents and they have learned if from *their* parents. Your early family life was one of limitation. You were controlled because you did not know what was good for you. Your parents believed that control and close supervision would prevent injuries from occurring. You developed your own belief in control.

The root of control is fear. When danger lurks behind every bush, control seems like the only thing that will work. Through awareness, understanding, and insight, you create change. Life is meant to be joyful and fulfilling. You have the right to experience your life as a movable feast, not a faithless journey of struggle and sickness.

When I first met Patricia, she was in law enforcement and wanted to change the type of work she was doing. She felt it was very unsuited for her nature. She was slight of build and not very tall, yet she found herself battling with drug addicts and alcoholics as part of her daily routine. What was keeping her stuck in her job and unable to change was that she had been abused as a child. As a result, she needed to control her life. As a police officer, she was in control. Subsequently, she was able to release her need for control and moved on.

What you experience is the result of your inner landscape. Even the work you do or the career you choose will represent your inner world. The number of people in law enforcement who have been sexually abused is a greater percentage than the civilian population. One of the symptoms of sexual abuse is the need for control. Drug and alcohol abuse are another attempt at controlling your inner world. Reformed alcoholics often become control addicts. They have given up their alcohol addiction for yet another addiction.

Remember, your ego is completely invested in control. It believes that control can work and it will move heaven and earth to prove it, no matter what the cost. You think that by applying more control, you will get a better result, but it only leads to creating more of what you *don't* want. This can become a never-ending cycle. The act of

control interferes with the natural flow of the universe and
its innate intelligence.

# # #

CHAPTER EIGHT
TRUSTING LIFE

When you trust life, the door is open for things to happen that are beyond your current comprehension. Whether you find your inspiration from Buddhism, the Bible, Kabbalah, or the Qur'an, you will ultimately find that when you combine trust with faith, self-awareness expands.

In a sense, you have been brainwashed into believing in control and predictability. In truth, you have another option available. Faith propels the energy of change. This is a great leap to take, as you have been conditioned to believe that the future is threatening. Your task is to dissociate from that belief. It is entirely up to you to make the effort, to step back from your conditioning and decide for yourself what the truth really is.

Peace, well-being, and fulfillment are entirely up to you. They are your birthright; they are buried under many layers of conditioning, but they are your true nature. You find those qualities through acceptance, not fighting with what happens to you. When you say no to what you are experiencing, you create more suffering. Acceptance brings peace.

The truth is subtle. In the world you live in, you have been conditioned to respond to messages that override your senses. Sometimes you completely miss anything that isn't louder than the chatter of the ego. Commercials on television are always louder than the program itself. Marketing executives know that in order to get your attention, they have to overwhelm you. Network programmers know full well, perhaps too well, the value of shock. Truth, however, comes from that quiet place within. That place where silence is the backdrop for the wisdom of your Higher Nature.

The future has been and always will be unknown. The entire culture and its institutions want to make sure you look to them for security. When you know that you will always be safe, you can stop giving up your sovereignty. In a world where there is constant change brought on by modern technology, philosophical, and cultural shifts, the truth is often hard to discern. As change accelerates, it tends to create chaos and anxieties.

To let go and accept where you are in your life may seem extremely difficult right now. Perhaps once you get to a better place in your life, it will be easier, but that time and place may never arrive. As you accept and replace the anxiety of not knowing, with trust, it will gradually become easier and easier to accept what is, and experience peace.

Virtually no one in this society or in any Western culture trusts life. Everyone locks their doors, and builds barricades against intrusion by savages. Anyone, and everyone, who believes they will be violated, will be. When you begin to truly believe you are safe, you create a different life dynamic.

Pete was a recovering alcoholic. When I met him, he had lost everything: his money, his family, his job—all was lost to alcohol and drugs. His guilt and his fear about his situation were overwhelming. I encouraged him to meditate and pray, something that he had never done before. He had never had any spiritual training, and he said he was not even sure he believed there was a God. I taught him the simple meditation techniques in Chapter One. He earned money by panhandling, slept at a mission at night, and he felt only despair and hopelessness. His only place to meditate was on a park bench near the Pike Place Market in downtown Seattle. It wasn't far from where he slept at night, but it was quiet in comparison to the noise of the shelter.

Through his prayer and meditation, his trust and faith began to grow. He expressed his feeling that something dramatic was going to happen, although he said that he had no idea what it would be. One day while he was meditating on the bench, a man stopped to talk to him. He told Pete he had seen him out there every day and that he suspected Pete was not sleeping, but was meditating. The man said that he was a Buddhist and meditated in his office every day at lunch. He invited Pete to a Buddhist meditation. A few days after attending the meditation, the man offered Pete a job working in a warehouse which his company owned. Pete accepted, and now two years later, he is a shift foreman, who meditates every day during his lunch hour.

When your fear is not blocking the doorway, synchronicity can come into your life. The universe will martial its forces to assist you in creating a new reality. Teachers, books, tools, and insights will come to you. The message and messenger will arrive.

As a business man, I would have been more successful had I been aware of the subtle truths and messages that were constantly coming to me. Almost everything being done in the business world today is still governed by control and personal will. To the ordinary business manager, surrendering and relinquishing the iron fist of control takes a leap of faith that few are willing to risk. They are mostly still depending on mission statements and time management techniques to arrive at their goals. If you surrender and let go, the results will show up before you can even set your goals.

Humans feel separate from everyone and everything in their world. That belief in separation creates a lack of trust, and disconnects you from the wisdom of the universe. Humanity separated from its Higher Nature thousands of years ago. The Old Testament talks about this in Genesis. It is called "the fall," or "separation," and occurred when Adam and Eve ate the forbidden fruit from the tree of knowledge of good and evil. The Greeks began to separate Spirit from matter in their writings around 500 B.C. and it has been with us since then.

There are 300 million people in the United States. Imagine what would happen if everyone chose to completely trust and integrate with their Higher Nature. Trust reconnects you with everything, including the planet itself. Most people do not realize that they are connected to the planet and all other life forms. Through your connection to the earth, you begin to restore balance. The separation you perceive is pure fallacy. God, the forest, even trees, can and do speak to you. It is only because of your beliefs that you do not hear them.

There is a city park in Seattle called Green Lake. As I was walking around the lake one blustery spring morning, a tree spoke to me. "Preposterous!" I can hear you say. "Trees don't talk." Well, I didn't know they could talk either, until that windy day in March. Green Lake is about four miles north of downtown Seattle, just west of the I-5 freeway. It's a city park occupying about one square mile of land. It's an idyllic spot landscaped with shrubs and huge oak trees, lots of plants, and a few evergreens. It boasts an on-site, indoor Olympic-sized swimming pool. The lake itself is rather shallow and is perfect for the hundreds of resident ducks and geese that call it home. It's a convenient place for the migrating Canadian geese to stop for a rest as they recuperate and head south for the winter. On the downside, the lake becomes somewhat polluted, because of the droppings left behind by our feathery friends. There is continuous controversy around what can be done to thin their population.

An asphalt path about three miles in length, circles the lake. It is available year-round for eager skate boarders, bicyclers, joggers, and the people who enjoy a casual stroll. There are well-used tennis courts and lots of Frisbee players, crisscrossing the green lawns surrounding the lake. It's a wonderful place to play and exercise. You can even rent canoes or attend an outdoor theater at the southwest corner of the park.

Back to my "talking tree" story: As I walked past a huge one-hundred plus year-old oak tree, it said "I am sick." There was no mistaking the message; it was loud and clear. I instantly paused, walked up to it, leaned in close, and looked up its huge trunk. I wondered why it had spoken to me. In retrospect, I suppose it's because it knew I could hear the message without doubting its authenticity.

At the time, I lived about three miles north of the lake and had bicycled there to spend a relaxing morning cycling around it. After arriving back home, I eagerly called a friend to share what had happened earlier; I knew she would be receptive to my experience. As I was talking, she turned to her three year-old son and told him that a tree had spoken to me. His immediate response was to deny that trees could talk. Amazing! At only three years of age, he had already taken on the cultural limitation that only *humans* can speak to humans.

Everything is conscious and therefore capable of communicating with humans if they want to, and if we are receptive. Sadly, most people remain closed to the possibility of nature communicating with humans. Why should they even *try* to speak to us, when so few are listening and capable of hearing the message?

When I told my friend, Lori, the story of the sick tree, not only was she receptive, she quickly suggested we go to Green Lake because she knew what to do to help the tree. After I pointed out the tree, she began circling it and chanting a strange language that seemed somehow familiar to me. Later on, I realized it was very similar to the deva language I had heard while in Thailand. The deva language is used by indigenous healers all over the globe. It is a kind of chant that wells up from deep within, and assists them in the healing process. Now, many years later, I'm happy to report the tree is still alive and well.

It was late spring and there were still clumps of snow on the ground, covered with pine needles and other debris. Richard Krull and I had decided to go to Denny Creek in the foothills of the Cascade Mountains. Richard is a man who wears the shirt of mysticism as he moves through life, and he's very sensitive and aware of just how alive and conscious the earth really is.

We walked along the mile-long trail next to the creek, winding through the forest and up to the bottom of beautiful Franklin Falls. It plummets over a sheer, granite-faced cliff and drops about 1,500 feet into Denny Creek. As we approached the waterfall, I asked Richard, "Can you feel that presence?"

"Yes," he said, "It feels as though a mist has settled in around us."

"Do you know what it is?" I asked.

Richard grew quiet and looked around us, a distant look in his eyes. "It's the consciousness of Denny Creek and the land around us."

"What does it want?" I inquired.

"I'm not sure," Richard replied, "But let's sit on that log over there and I'll see if it can speak to me."

Sitting on a moss-covered log under the canopy of branches provided by the trees, Richard blended in with and become part of the landscape. He was deeply absorbed and in communion with the forest and the land.

"I am indeed the consciousness of this land," it said through Richard. "This land is a sacred place that has been violated by man. It was an ancient burial site for the Native population who once lived in these parts. When the White man came here, he paid little attention to the sacredness of the area or to the spiritual customs of the people who lived here for many years. You can do little about that.

"Over the past one hundred years—since this area was logged and clear-cut—it has become a park, a place to come and explore nature, rest and relax, and become more attuned to the trees and the fauna at the edge of the creek.

"The creek is the result of a great subterranean pool that lies beneath these mountains. It is part of what you call your watershed."

"What can we do to help people understand that the earth and the land are sacred, conscious organisms?" I asked.

"Help establish more awareness of your connection to the earth. You do not understand that you are part of the planetary system, as much so as the trees and the rocks, rivers, and oceans. Assist people in the realization that the earth is alive and must be treated with love and respect. Bring others to this location to share this experience with you. Even those who are already trying to clean up your waste have little understanding of how alive and aware I really am."

It was very still. The only other sound I could hear was the gurgling and splashing of the creek as it sped on down the mountain.

Richard breathed deeply and began again.

"My message to you is that you have too long neglected your home and soiled your nest. But it is not too late to correct what you have done." Richard began to speak haltingly, "The oceans, the forest lands. They are resilient. If you begin now in earnest to save the environment, the planet can be saved."

Another unusual experience I had was when I saw a dragon, while meditating in a cave in northern Thailand. The cave is a fairly typical large cave for Thailand. It goes back into the hillside about three-quarters of a mile. It has thirty-foot-high ceilings, bats, and places where if you make the wrong turn you may never be seen again (a fate not so long ago, of a German tourist). The cave is dark, damp, and a little smelly. Numerous monks have used it as a place of refuge to meditate and pray. Near the back of the cave, there is a stairway to the lower level. The stairway is so steep it might as well be a ladder. There is actually another level even lower than the one the stairs lead to. When I was there, it was filled with water left over from the rainy season. The lowest level is reported to be the home of the Chiang Dow Dragon. I was somewhat skeptical that such a dragon existed; no doubt the Thai version of Bigfoot or the Loch Ness monster.

A group of us who were on a month-long meditation retreat went to tour the cave, which is also used as a Buddhist temple by the local villagers. It is quite a picturesque place, nestled in the arms of a heavily forested mountain, near the Burmese border. We were led through the cave and its many passages by three young Thais with battery-powered lanterns. At one point during our tour, we had to get down on our hands and knees and crawl through a narrow passage for about ten feet to get to another part of the cave. The narrow passage is the only way you can get to the lower level where the dragon is reported to be. Water seeped from the walls of the cave in many areas and it smelled of bat guano. Many of us carried flashlights and by pointing them upward, we could see the bats on the ceilings.

I took a seat on a bench that had been carved out of stone. By that time, we were very experienced meditators and had spent nearly a month in deep meditation. A typical day for us was to get up at 5 a.m. and spend the next twelve hours in meditation with a forty-five minute break for lunch and then back into meditation. Sometimes we would meditate all night long without sleeping. One of the reasons for going there was to meditate in the absolute silence of the cave.

Within moments, I slipped into a deep, meditative state. Almost immediately, I heard what sounded like a cough, but it didn't seem human. A chill ran up my spine as I wondered where the sound had come from. I thought I felt a presence. I opened my eyes but nothing was there. Quickly, I closed my eyes again and then I heard a distinctive roar. There was no mistaking the sound for anything but the roar of a dragon or maybe a stray tiger, which was even *less* likely, because there aren't any wild tigers left in Southeast Asia.

Suddenly, standing directly in front of me, was the Chiang Dao Dragon. He looked like any other dragon you might see painted on the wall of a Chinese temple, with a face like a lion, sporting horns and massive claws. He was a ferocious looking beast, yet love radiated from his eyes.

Startled, I opened my eyes and he was gone. I'd also heard the voice of another dragon, an infant. No one had mentioned the existence of a baby dragon, but later on I found out that it had also been heard by others. I closed my eyes and the Chiang Dow Dragon was back, almost immediately. I get it, I thought to myself. This beast lives in another dimension and I can only see him when I am meditating; while in meditation, I often transcend dimensions. It's been said that he sometimes manifests into this dimension where *we* are.

No doubt, many people will reject this out of hand as fantasy. I could have chosen to believe it was simply a hallucination of some sort, but that choice would have limited my future experiences. It is faith that opens you to the experiences that will reconnect you to the wisdom of Higher Nature, and your link to all life on this dimension and others.

In order to regain trust, you must be open to the possibility that there is life beyond your present awareness. That part of you that you call ego absolutely does not want anything to do with experiences beyond your five senses. It is totally invested in the status quo. It wants you to operate as you always have. How often do you go over the same ground, rehashing the same problems over and over and attracted to the same types of relationships again and again? You may not enjoy being stuck in the same job or the same old relationship, but it is familiar ground. In order to create change, you must trust that something better will come along, and rely on the Divine intelligence that created you.

Children are naturally spontaneous and trusting, but as they grow, limits are placed on what is acceptable. The result is the loss of faith in their own experiences. Certain actions are not accepted as "normal" by adults, so in order to please your role models and peers, you learned as a child, to disregard who you *really* are, in favor of a more "acceptable" version. An experienced psychoanalyst once commented to me that children are always curious about life, yet he rarely observed that quality in his adult clients. Spontaneity and curiosity invariably lead to experiences that are beyond the five senses and even paranormal experiences. Of course, children are frequently ridiculed for believing such experiences are real. Often people try to allow just enough awareness into their lives so they can get from one point to another—guarded awareness, it might be called. Limiting parts of your experience disconnects you from the wisdom of the universe. There is an old saying, "Go within, or go without." What will you find within? You will find the wisdom of the universe.

Those of you in business may be thinking that all of this is fine and dandy for the average person, but in no way are you going to trust the universe to make a good sports shoe, tennis racket, or even a Frisbee. Most business people are highly stressed, because they are trying to do everything on their own. Business managers would do much better if they would meditate a few minutes each day and ask for guidance. Solutions will come to you if you have faith. Faith is the crucible of change, the alchemy of your Higher Nature.

In his book *Conversations with God,* Neale Donald Walsch addresses this issue by stating that God is always talking to you. The question is not whether God is speaking to you, but whether or not you are listening. You may not actually hear the voice of the universe speaking words in your head; it may communicate through what you see or what other people say or do. Your soul knows truth. In fact, it knows *only* truth. Certainly, some time in our past, humans knew the truth of their existence. Even today there are isolated groups or tribes of people who know the truth. A popular book entitled *Mutant Message Down Under,* by Marlo Morgan, describes a small tribe of aborigines who live their lives in complete trust of the universe. They were nomads, who survived in a vast desert, without tools or any other modern convenience. Everything is scarce where they live, especially food and water. They arise every morning with little in the way of supplies and they pray for guidance. Every day, all of their needs are somehow fulfilled. They are safe, and they are supported, in the middle of nowhere, where everything is scarce. If you had no food every morning when you awoke, and there were no restaurants or stores, what would you do? Most of you would not survive. Those people have survived for centuries by believing and trusting that they would be taken care of, that their needs would be met, which they are.

Trust implies having faith in something greater and wiser than yourself. You are not alone, abandoned to the vagrancies of this world like a ship without a rudder. Your

Higher Nature is constantly speaking to you in one way or another, through feeling, synchronicity, coincidence, and frequently through other people. A constant barrage of symbols are warning you, and guiding you, to a future of health and well-being. A mustard seed does not require proof that the sun is shining, before it begins to stretch toward the sunlight.

# # #

CHAPTER NINE
RELATIONSHIPS

Every relationship in your life is colored by the single most important relationship you have—your relationship with your Higher Nature, or God. You are really two selves—The Little Self, or ego, and the Big Self, which is your Higher Nature. Self-awareness comes from the Big Self.

Most people are totally identified with the Little Self. The division between ego and the Big Self creates opposition. This separation between the two selves creates the fear and insecurity you experience. You are the Big Self. The Little Self is false, a make-believe self that you have become identified with. Why *wouldn't* you believe it's who you are, when that is the only thing you know?

For almost everyone, relationships create the most significant polarity of all. You cannot possibly feel secure when you believe that you are separate from your Higher Nature. It is the source of primal pain and fear, the reason life appears to be so threatening.

Life itself poses no threat. All conflict is simply a reflection of your belief that you are separate. The Big Self is the source of life. The Little Self is a paper tiger, created by identifying with mind and thought. You think that a larger home, more money in your bank account, or a new car, will make you more complete and secure. But you have found the ego's appetite to be insatiable. All of your political and religious structures are an attempt to bridge the distance you perceive between the Little Self and your Higher Nature. Throughout history, there have been great teachings that have attempted to explain the oneness of creation, but few have taken them seriously. Any religion that doesn't teach you that you and your Higher Nature are one is not a true religion.

The physical universe was created by what is commonly known as the "Big Bang!" Though you may think of it as a huge explosion, in actuality, the event was more like a spectacular cosmic "expansion." Have you ever wondered what was there before that event? Astronomers and physicists suggest that there was *nothing* there. At the point of the big bang, that "nothing" became "something," and for whatever reason, God decided to take "form." He didn't just *create* the universe, He *became* the universe.

Mythology, rituals, and symbolism abound in an attempt to increase your understanding of your relationship with the Big Self, or God. Yet, the masses remain confused and insecure in their knowledge of their true nature. Over the next decade or so, there will be a massive shift in understanding your spiritual nature. If this doesn't happen, the earth will cease to exist.

The disease you experience, or even the stress you feel, is the result of the disconnect from who you really are; I said this earlier in the book. Your Higher Nature, or awareness, is the healing force of the universe. A recent medical study shows that 56 percent of the doctors in the study believe that spirituality and religion have a significant influence on healing. The percentage of the doctors who believe that spirituality and religion help people cope with illness is approximately 76 percent. Accelerated healing occurs as you become aware of your connection to the Big

Self. The universe is self-correcting. So, even without any awareness, you might experience some healing. "Wow!" I hear you say, "I don't really have to take responsibility for my own healing." But before you begin to celebrate, you might want to think about this. Even if you manage to heal your cancer or other life-threatening disease, it will very likely come back even stronger than before. Where there is no self-awareness, there will never be significant, permanent healing.

It is the Little Self that wants to keep you in the dark and away from the light of self-awareness. It can't stand the idea of giving up its role as captain of the Titanic, even when it knows the ship is going to sink; ego is in charge, for better or for worse. In fact, ego often approves of an experience, even when it knows it will be harmful, because that strengthens its identity.

In order to heal your relationships with other people, you have to see the big picture and look for a way to heal the relationship with your Higher Nature. In truth, there is only one life form on the planet. It looks like there are many others, but that's just a perception created by the Little Self. Oneness is not just an idea; it's the way it is. You are simply not aware of unity and the Little Self wants to keep it that way. Integration with the Big Self certainly is no small task in a culture, which to a large extent, hides from, ignores, and even denies its own spirituality. Denying who you are immediately blunts any attempt to rectify the problem. Some religions and those who claim to have direct contact with God, purposely keep you from a personal relationship with Him. This is a convenient way for those who see themselves as ordained, to make the case that ordinary men do not have the ability to experience their own divinity.

Many religions believe they have the only access point to God, and that their way is the only way, but it is the Little Self that takes that stance. Even the Constitution of the United States says, "All men are created equal." Acceptance is a quality of your Higher Nature and it doesn't see anyone, or anything, as inferior; intolerance is ego. Believing your thoughts are real and have meaning, leads to intolerance and creates a hierarchy. Thought separates you from your Higher Nature and as far as the Little Self is concerned, that's okay; it's just fine.

For centuries, those who tried to bypass the church and create an open door to God have been persecuted, tortured, and dismembered by the high priests of organized religion. Of course, the collective psyche maintains this memory and is deterred by it, albeit not consciously.

It is your relationship with your Higher Nature which sets the stage for all of your other relationships. Many therapists believe that no other issue really matters, but they are still in the minority. They believe that restoring your connection to your Higher Nature and realizing who you really are can heal your issues. No doubt this is true, but most of you will benefit by taking smaller steps first. Healing the separation between you and your Higher Nature is the goal. But you will probably have to start with more peripheral issues like healing your relationship with your parents, spouse, children, and others. All of these issues are a warm-up, preparation for healing the biggest wound of all—your belief in separation between the Little Self and the Big Self.

Western cultures have become more secular since the industrial revolution, and even more so since you began to rely on science to solve your problems. This is especially a twentieth century phenomenon. Science began to dominate Western cultures at the turn of the twentieth century when it took the place of spirituality and God.

As the twenty-first century unfolds, there is even more emphasis on science. Technology has begun to marry with biology and promises to extend life. Many believe this will lead to less disease and a longer life, but science and technology are false Gods. Biological life allows your Higher Nature to experience the physical world. Biological life is actually an illusion, like a symbolic dream. The Little Self wants to make it real and meaningful. Dr. Albert Einstein expressed it like this: "Reality is merely an illusion, albeit a persistent one." The Vedas, Buddhism, and even many quantum physicists, agree that life is an illusion.

A Course in Miracles says, "Nothing real can be threatened." In other words, the finite cannot, in any way, affect the infinite. It also says, "Nothing unreal exists." This means that anything with a beginning, middle, and an ending, isn't real. It doesn't actually exist; it's merely an illusion. Making the illusion real creates more suffering and struggle.

Your biological parents are merely caretakers for this lifetime. You may have had hundreds, even thousands, of biological caretakers throughout your incarnations. Every incarnation puts you together with a new set of biological parents, however, souls tend to reincarnate within the same grouping. There was a classic example of this with a group of people in a small town in Nevada who had memories of living together in the south, during the Civil War. Those people appeared on local and national television. The evidence they presented was very compelling. No doubt you have been with your parents before. You, in your wisdom, selected the parents who would best facilitate the experiences you need in this lifetime. If you have trouble believing you've had other lifetimes, it really doesn't matter. Take away from this discussion what feels right to you. At a later date, you may embrace these ideas—or not.

By turning within and listening carefully, you can determine what your Higher Nature desires for you. When you begin to understand that the life you are experiencing is completely of your own choosing, there is often confusion and bewilderment. Why would anyone choose a lifetime with such pain, sickness, and suffering? If life were your choice, certainly you would choose something else. Many a sage has tried to explain the reasoning behind the choices you make: to balance karma, to experience duality, to discover who you are as well as who you are not, to name a few. On the surface, it may appear as if you have made some kind of mistake by picking a lifetime as difficult as this one. But your search for healing has brought you to this information. It increases your understanding of how disease is created and allows you to begin healing and growing. It is virtually impossible for you to see the big picture as long as you are separated from the wisdom of your Higher Nature.

It is the movement away from pain and suffering, toward healing, peace, and wisdom, that has brought you here. It may look like you are being punished by a vengeful God, when actually you are being given the gift of finding grace amongst the rubble and chaos of your life. It is out of your identification with mind, thought, and ego, that you have become stuck in suffering. Surrender to who you are, and you will move into that place of grace and well-being. Healing and finding grace are the same things. Grace is simply a little further along on the path of healing. Pain is the greatest teacher.

To survive this life with ease, you must learn to live without judgment. You must be in that place of balance where there are no opposites. Many of you, who read this book and heal your malady, will go almost immediately back to your old paradigm without giving any thought to the idea that you are actually your Higher Nature, disguised as a human. If you give in to your Little Self's desire to dominate your life, you will find yourself continuing to blame others for what you experience and you will begin suffering; again, your cancer or other disease will likely return. This is another wake up call. Your Higher Nature is telling you to wake up and acknowledge who you are.

Integrating with the Big Self may be as simple as beginning to meditate. It will include an exploration of your psychological issues, because they prevent self-awareness. Your exploration will begin to loosen the denial that creates the split between the Little Self and the Big Self. For reasons that never really make any sense, many people find looking at their issues to be very difficult. The initial resistance is often in deference to your parents. In a sense, you have formed a pact with your parents to keep them from being exposed. It is hard for you to admit that your parents were wrong, but it's really your ego's resistance to change that creates the dilemma. Ridiculous as it may seem, honoring this deception has kept humanity bound to the wheel of pain and suffering for centuries. The truth will set you and every member of your family free, including those who have passed on.

An entire industry has grown up around counseling. Many therapists are trying to teach their clients how to cope with physical reality and assist them in making better decisions. There are many skills you can learn which are useful. They will assist you with the issues you experience in your life and in your relationships. The awareness created by exploring your unconscious mind will begin to allow the light of truth into the deepest recesses of your mind. Therapy may begin to restore your primary relationship with the Big Self.

I spent many years in psychoanalysis and have participated in many modalities of self-exploration and healing. They are all useful, but for many, they tend to be Band-Aids and may just disguise the real problem. My psychoanalyst was the first person to discuss spiritual matters with me. He realized that ultimately you all have to embrace your spirituality if you are to grow and heal. Without understanding the nature of your spirituality, you will always feel lost. As long as you identify with your mind and thoughts, you will feel alone and abandoned, and will continue to suffer and struggle. The pain you experience can destroy you and the world you live in. As your awareness and connection to your Big Self increases, you become more integrated and will stop suffering.

This cannot be overstated. You are addicted to the idea that your mind and thoughts are who you are. You have all seen a person walking along a crowded street, talking incessantly out loud; you think they are insane! They are obviously identified with what they are saying, even though to you, it's absolute nonsense. Actually, they are reflecting your own nonsensical inner voice. It's just that you don't speak your thoughts out loud. You are just as addicted to the chatter as they are. It creates the intense pain and suffering you experience. Your addiction to mind and thought creates disease and can kill you.

Your personal suffering and inability to find peace in relationships is a result of the disconnect from your Higher Nature. As you practice the simple techniques in this book, you will become more integrated and begin to realize your true nature. Your ego will try to discount what I have said. It will try to denigrate what has been presented here; it will fight to survive. Ego is very clever.

The most basic communication skill you have is the capacity to be a good listener. People love a good listener, a person who doesn't tune them out or who is just waiting for the chance to tell their own personal story. Most people are not good listeners because their own issues rise to the surface as soon as you begin to speak. It is impossible for you to be a good listener if your own unconscious mind is a garbage can full of fear, anger, and other issues. If you are having trouble with the message in this chapter, it is because it's in conflict with your ego's agenda and its fight for survival.

To listen is the greatest service you can offer another. Listen to them and hear what they have to say.

Listen with your entire being. You will not be able to receive love if you cannot listen. You serve your Higher Nature by listening. Something else you gain through listening is clarity around your own issues. The person in your life telling you about their problems is reflecting your own issues back to you. The likelihood that they are in your life, without sharing similar issues, is nil. They are in your life because you share a similar emotional pathology. They are there as an outer reflection of your inner landscape.

To most people, sex does not seem very Godly or spiritual. The idea that some things are divine and some are not, is simply another polarity. God does not make judgments about sexuality. Obviously, sexuality is God given. Humans certainly did not create it. You have been taught that sex is not love. That simply is not true, except when it is sought after out of fear, anger, or a feeling of incompleteness. Sexual union is perhaps one of the few times you actually feel connected to someone else. This creates another paradox: The more disconnected you are from your Higher Nature, the less connected you can be with anyone else, sexually or otherwise.

Morality is in the eye of the beholder. Sexual mores continuously change. For instance, there are societies in North America who believe in non-monogamous lifestyles. The founders of the Mormon Church believed in polygamy; it was acceptable for a man to have several wives. Though it is illegal, polygamy is still alive and well in the United States. Most people believe you should be faithful to your partner, but is that not ownership and control of someone else's sexuality? A clue to what's going on when your partner is unfaithful is in your response, "What's wrong with me?" As you heal your own relationship with your Higher Nature, you will begin to see the truth for yourself.

Sex is really just another human experience. Some religions have injected their beliefs into the rightness and wrongness of sexuality. They think they know what is right for someone else, but their ignorance is plain to see. Only you can determine what is right or wrong for you. Anyone who thinks they have the answer for others is simply deceiving themselves.

Though I believe you should honor your agreements with your partner or spouse, most of all, you must stop judging yourself and others, whatever the circumstances. Of course, that is one of the hardest things to do. When you stop judging yourself, you will stop judging others. Maybe it cannot be done in a human body, but certainly you can do a better job than you have been doing. There is always room for improvement.

Isn't it interesting that communication and sexuality are two of the most significant human issues you have to cope with, yet they are probably the most confusing and distorted of all human behavior. There are many issues that can separate you from your Higher Nature, but separation is not its choice. If you see God as vengeful and judgmental, then you will want to hide your issues. The view that God believes in retribution is the result of projecting human qualities onto God. Judgment is based in fear and is strictly a human quality. Healing the division between the Little Self and the Big Self can be as simple as using the breath technique. Your belief in separation is the cause of your maladies and suffering. It is the primary cause of your feelings of abandonment and betrayal. If you were completely integrated with the Big Self, you could not become sick.

The Vedas say that the finite cannot understand the infinite. All of the spiritual teachings that I am aware of, agree with The Vedas. Even the Bible says that man cannot totally understand God.

The Tao Te Ching was written by Lao Tzu, about 2,600 years ago, in China, and is one of the world's most profound spiritual books. It says, "The Tao that can be spoken is not the true Tao." The wisdom of God cannot be put into words. Words do not, and cannot, describe God. God speaks to you through your feelings; it's the reason you need to restore your ability to "feel." He also speaks to you through impressions, inspiration, intuition, and visions. Some suggest that God is love, but no one really knows what that means, or what love actually is. Ego is fear-based and fear and love are opposites. As long as you are identified with ego, there is little room for love. With most people, love is conditional, therefore it isn't true love. Joy is very close to love, but who is joyful all of the time? No one.

The first time I mentioned to Susan that most people are angry with God and feel abandoned by their creator, she vehemently stated that she knew God had not abandoned her. Intellectually, Susan believed that God had not abandoned her, but I sensed she was not being truthful and was in denial of her real feelings. Working with clients has shown me that you are very likely in denial of your anger toward God. Why do so many people deny their anger? Because many religions teach that God will punish you for your thoughts. Susan's response had seemed very mental, without feeling and conviction. Then one day during a session, she became aware of her own anger toward God for abandoning her. That revelation brought about an eruption of painful feelings which lasted for an hour. Then, a strange thing happened in her relationship with her partner. She grew closer to him and their communication greatly improved. This was a result of her healing her relationship with God, and therefore with herself and her partner. Instead of harboring thoughts of leaving her current relationship, she began to create the change she desired.

It is possible for you to return to your natural state of grace, wisdom, and love. You may have to make this journey one step at a time, but even that isn't all bad. **The lessons learned one step at a time will certainly never** be forgotten, and you will have no need to repeat them in the future.

# # #

CHAPTER TEN
Life Purpose

Most people wonder if they are living a purposeful life. The answer is yes. All lives reflect purpose. Becoming more integrated with your Higher Nature will reveal a higher purpose, and believe it or not, your illness is part of that purpose; it motivates you to explore who you are and causes you to look within for healing.

The dissatisfaction you feel is telling you that something more satisfying is available to you. The path to a more fulfilling life demands two things: a strong connection to your Higher Nature so that it can better guide you, and clearing obstacles that are keeping you from healing and evolving. Something more fulfilling is available to anyone who is willing to do those two things.

Purpose can be divided into two categories—higher, or inner purpose, and outer purpose. Your inner purpose is to reintegrate with your Higher Nature and live from that vantage point. In that regard, your dissatisfaction is your greatest ally, because it causes you to turn inward. There is really no other way to create change. The outer purpose is what you do in the material world. It too, will change as you become more integrated.

The stronger your connection to your Higher Nature, the greater your ability is to create change. The mind cannot create change. Only your Higher Nature can do that. Your outer purpose isn't static and as you grow and evolve, it will morph into something new. What you believe it to be in your twenties may be very different in your thirties or forties, and it can change dramatically in your fifties. You are half way through life, maybe a little more. Your values begin to shift and change, often from the materialistic, to a more inward view. Your children are gone and your life as a homemaker or head of household is no longer as important. This allows you more time to explore the depth of life.

To find meaning and satisfaction in this lifetime, you will have to come into alignment with your inner and outer purpose. One of the most rewarding things you can do is to fulfill your higher purpose. Your illness is related to purpose; it is indeed, integral to the process of self-discovery. If you are not growing and evolving, you will feel stuck and out of alignment with life.

Many people spend a great deal of their lives searching for purpose, claiming all the while if only they could *find* it, they would be happy. Even though you say you want to discover your purpose, you may be unwilling to face the change it will entail. What many people are really looking for is a way to satisfy their ego's version of what *it* thinks it needs to be happy. This is usually a far cry from what your soul wants, and chances are, it does not include a lot of change. If finding purpose means dramatic change, there will be a lot of resistance to finding it.

As I said earlier, it takes courage to change, because it requires you to stop blaming others for the circumstances in your life. You may be reading this book because of an illness or because you are interested in prevention, but whether you know it or not, there is something else going on. You have come to this information, because you have felt the subtle breeze of the unknown and perhaps unknowable presence of your Higher Nature, entering your life. If you are like I was, you may not recognize that you are being ever so gently turned into the "winds of change." The reason for the subtlety is because, as you know, ego always resists change. A forceful shove would bring up a lot of its resistance. There are exceptions of course. Some people about to take this step will feel like they are being pushed off a cliff and will not survive. You may not be aware of how much your ego resists. As you make this journey of healing and growth, you will stretch the boundaries of your beliefs about the nature of reality. As you begin to explore the reality of your soul and Higher Nature, you will find that *nothing* is as it seems.

So, what are you looking for and why are you looking for it? Again, dissatisfaction with the status quo is the reason you or anyone else looks for change, and in this regard, dissatisfaction, even if it is the result of a debilitating disease, is your greatest ally. Without it, why would you want to alter your course? You wouldn't. For an alcoholic who finds himself passed out and face down in a dark alley, it is about physical survival. He will die if he doesn't change his ways. For you, it may be a disease or be less dramatic, but nevertheless, you are looking in a different direction than you would normally look, for fulfillment, satisfaction, and healing.

The reasons for wanting to take a different direction with your life may vary from person to person, but you know in your heart that you have been lied to all of your life and you want to know what the "truth" actually is. Everyone eventually comes to this point in one lifetime or another. You are at that point now, or you wouldn't have picked up this book and started to read it.

The mystery of life persists. You come and you go, and for those few short years you are here, you struggle to survive and find your way. The meaning of life remains obscure, for most. Most people struggle and suffer throughout life, knowing all along that it doesn't have to be that way. Many become addicted to struggle, and like any addiction, it defines their lives.

Many look to the physical world for fulfillment, yet as you look around, you'll find few, if any, who have found lasting peace or fulfillment in the material world. It may *look* like some have. Business tycoons and rock stars are paraded before us on the nightly talk shows as examples of the good life, but many of them succumb to drugs and alcohol. Their relationships don't work, and they are miserable and sick, yet many still seek fulfillment in "things." You know that none of this will bring you what you really desire, but you might be drawn to try "just one more time" to find what you are looking for, in the "stuff" the world has to offer. You may think a new relationship will help, a bigger house, a new car, maybe even a sports car. A better education might just do the trick. You go back to school to update your education and skills, and then join the rat race of the corporate world. You discover that striving creates a lot more stress than you had bargained for, and then you become ill. Many who fall down this rabbit hole are unable to climb back up, and will succumb to a lifetime of struggle, suffering, illness, or even death.

Most wealthy people will try to increase their wealth in order to enhance their feeling of security. This often leads to a never-ending cycle of accumulating more things. There is even a cultural expression that speaks to this: "The one who dies with the most toys wins." Those who think this way are truly lost.

I was watching The History Channel on TV one day. The story was about a man who had ordered an expensive, hand-made Bentley automobile, with a price tag of over $400,000. As the proud owner hobbled out of his mansion to take delivery of his new car, it was obvious that he was suffering from a severe, crippling disease. He must have believed that he would feel better by acquiring a new "thing" to placate his ego.

My own search for purpose and the meaning of life was the result of two decades of success and subsequent failures. I have always been an entrepreneur. By my late twenties, I was successful in business, however by my early thirties, I lost all that I had achieved. So, I hunkered down and found a regular job. Within a couple of years, I found a new avenue for my entrepreneurial flair and I became successful once more. Then, guess what happened? I *lost* it all again. By this time I had married and had a family to support. I was devastated by my losses and was very concerned for the security of my family. I began to experience a deep sense of insecurity, anxiety, and even depression. Of course those feelings had been there since early childhood, but they had been covered over by keeping busy, and of course, denial. One of the reasons everyone feels so much insecurity is because, as you know, ego is fear-based. Consequently, most people feel uneasy and insecure.

Because of my business failures and nagging anxieties, I decided to try psychotherapy as an avenue for exploring the reasons behind them. By that time, I had become addicted to prescription drugs and was drinking too much. While in therapy, I stopped drinking and taking tranquilizers. My anxieties diminished, but they didn't entirely disappear. My therapist explained that my anxieties were my ally, because they created the desire for a deeper exploration of who I was and what made me tick. Of course, I didn't really believe him at the time. Most people are looking for a quick fix, hence, the proliferation of psychiatric drugs. Often, an aggressive therapy for illnesses like cancer seems to work; a tumor may be eradicated, but it almost always comes back and is even more debilitating. This happens when you ignore the life changes you really need to make.

It can take a long time to unravel psychological issues that were acquired in early childhood, but if they are not cleared, they simply keep attracting their own likeness and drawing experiences to you that reinforce them.

As I progressed in therapy, I gained insight into how I responded to people and life situations. There were subtle shifts, but the underlying anxiety and stress did not totally abate.

My turn into the winds of change started in my forties. Prior to that, my entire focus had been on the "outer world" and how to make a buck. My attention was totally on the big three—sex, money, and power. Isn't that what all young men want? Though fame and power over others was never important to me, I certainly wanted money. Not just a little, but a lot of it. The same went for sex!

Most people think that having a lot of money will give them the security they desire, yet most never feel secure, no matter *how* much money they have. What you are really looking for is peace and fulfillment; it cannot be found in the accumulation of money and things. If you are sick, the first step is to get well, but if you ignore exploring your inner purpose, you will gain very little. The hole in your heart is created by not receiving enough love as a child, and it can never be filled by acquiring more "stuff."

Some people are incapable of turning inward, even for a moment. A certain amount of personal evolution is required before you can make that turn. It is the maturity of the individual's soul that makes it possible. It is usually the result of having many lifetimes here on earth, but the time it takes for that kind of maturation is becoming shorter, because the energies here on earth are shifting to a higher frequency. Ego can never become mature enough to make this transition, nor, does it actually want to. It's the individual soul that wants to make this transformation. The ego is too busy pretending to be in control of your life and chasing after the "big three." You can pat yourself on the back for being mature enough to turn inward. You draw this kind of information to you when you are ready to hear the message and not one moment sooner. If you were not capable of understanding and integrating this information, why would you attract it to yourself? You wouldn't. It's like the proverbial adage, "When the student is ready, the teacher will appear."

Crimes are committed every fifteen seconds here in the United States. So, how do those in authority respond? By spending more money, hiring more police, and making more laws. At the same time, individual citizens are installing burglar alarms and are arming themselves. It's obvious that none of these solutions are making you more secure. All of the news programs, talk shows, political pundits, politicians, and everyone with a microphone, are claiming that we are all victims of something, but your disease is the result of your inner programming. It looks like nothing is working; your world is out of control, and no matter how hard you try, nothing changes for the better. When was the last time you heard a politician or anyone in authority take responsibility for their own actions? This may be hard for you to swallow; it is one of the most mysterious and misunderstood aspects of life. Ultimately, it is you and *only* you who are responsible for your health, and everything else you experience.

There is no way you can change the outer world. You have already tried that with your spouse, partners, kids, and friends and it has been totally unsuccessful. As you know, you have to change your "inner" programming before you can stop attracting what you *don't* want into your life. But nothing will change if you continue to accept the world view that you are a victim.

Of course, your purpose may include an entire gestalt of qualities, a combination of potentials and skills found nowhere else on earth. This may seem far-fetched, but it is true. You are unique. There is no one like you on this planet or anywhere else in the entire universe. Nor, has there *ever* been someone exactly like you.

Growth is a never-ending process. Of course, it can look very different than you expect. You might even have to turn to the past in order to find what you are really looking for. I've worked with a number of clients who, because of parental or peer pressure, stopped pursuing something they found fulfillment in, as a child.

I suggested this to June, one of my young clients. She was almost immediately propelled back to childhood, when she had been very creative and excelled at crafts of all kinds. She had become quite skillful as a young artist and pottery maker. During puberty, however, her parents were not at all supportive. They told her she would never be able to make a living by becoming an artist. June gave up on her dreams and took on the belief that her parents had instilled. She subsequently went back to school and refined her artistic abilities. It didn't take long before she was able to build a successful career doing what she loved. Choosing to follow her original dream of becoming both an artist and potter was very fulfilling. If you don't get a big A-HA from reading this, then you probably need to spend time going inward and connecting with your Higher Nature.

Many people have discovered unknown qualities by meditating. Before I started clearing issues, beliefs, and old psychological patterns, I had no idea that I would eventually become a writer, therapist, and teacher.

John came to me because he was very dissatisfied with his job as a gardener. It didn't pay well enough, but he enjoyed it. During the course of his one-hour session, we learned that working as a gardener was indeed in line with his purpose in this lifetime. His purpose was to cultivate a deep connection with the earth, and he did this by gardening. One of the options he considered was working as a salesman for a wholesale gardening company. Doing so would keep him in touch with plants and the earth's energy. This would align with his evolving purpose for this lifetime, as well as afford him a better life.

Purpose is an integral part of your life; given even the slightest chance your purpose will find *you*. Being in alignment with your inner and outer purpose creates a life which is satisfying and fulfilling. As you evolve, your inner and outer purposes will merge. If you do not receive an adequate reward for what you are doing, something is wrong. Purpose always includes prosperity, or at least a comfortable living. This is to say, once you are fulfilling your purpose, you will realize that you will be supported and provided for.

Most people live compartmentalized lives. Work is one thing, play another, and relationships yet another. **When you are in alignment with your inner purpose, work becomes play, struggle ceases, and your life blossoms effortlessly. All of your activity becomes a communion with your Higher Nature, a demonstration of love, which adds a whole new dimension to the dance of your life.**

Finding purpose is simply discovering your own uniqueness. Whatever your contribution is intended to be, it will be a highly sought after quality, because only *you* will have that quality, knowledge, and ability. This is the one thing that makes you like no other. Some of these qualities will be obvious, if you give them some consideration. Others will be more obscure and you will have to go inward to find them. Your purpose may seem mundane. If it does, don't become discouraged. It's probably just an interim step. Once you realize why you are here, you will find that you are a highly creative person relative to your purpose. You will be filled with ideas and inspiration.

If everyone were to discover their own uniqueness and higher purpose, no one would be hungry, homeless, or unemployed. Humanity would evolve beyond imagination. As it is, many industries are stalled or failing. They cannot progress until the right person supplies them with some unique quality or information. That is how important your contribution can be. Every invention existed as an idea first.

Wherever you are right now, stop and consider the demonstration of individual purpose and creativity which makes up the modern world. The automobiles, microwave ovens, Teflon, Velcro, synthetics, vegetable oil, refrigeration, and every tool you utilize in your life, is the result of someone's unique contribution and purpose.

Your purpose is encoded in your DNA. You are not your ego and personality; that is simply the stance you are taking in this lifetime. You are your Higher Nature, disguised as a human. You have been created in the image and likeness of God, and inherent in that likeness is everything you need. This is not a new thought. It's been said for thousands of years, but like all simple truths, the meaning has been lost. If you can accept that your life has a higher purpose, then it follows that you also have the potential to actualize that purpose.

Successful people everywhere have used their individual uniqueness to build the foundations of their lives. A few years back, a neighbor and friend of mine had the unique ability to build small, wooden boats capable of holding only one or two fishermen. At that time, most boats were being made from fiberglass, but my friend's wooden boats were so much in demand that he couldn't build them fast enough. Even though he was retired, he found himself busier than ever—and absolutely loving it!

An inability to find purpose simply means you need to clear more obstacles. The complete picture might come to you all at once, or over a period of time. As you increase your awareness, your purpose will probably change course.

At some point in your evolution, your purpose will include stewardship of the planet. Everyone is connected to the planet in some way, but as you evolve, you become more aware of your connection to the planetary energy systems. Humans are inherently part of the ecosystem of the earth. You may not be aware of your role with the planet, but as you grow, it will emerge. We have come to an intersection in time on this planet, when it is not enough to simply deal with the human purpose on earth. Humanity is running out of time. You must learn to have a more universal view of life, and reconnect with your spiritual heritage.

Meditating for a few minutes each day will begin to re-establish your connection to your higher purpose. Your ego may put up a ferocious struggle to put forth its own agenda. Your Higher Nature will wait until you surrender and let go of your past, and then drop a new blueprint into place. You will find your life's work when you are willing to give up your preconceived ideas as to what it ought to look like. It can look like almost anything. You might be here to experience power or service, such as a Bill Gates, Bill Clinton, or perhaps a Mother Teresa. She lived without worldly goods. John was a gardener because his life purpose was to learn about the earth. You will discover that your purpose and blueprint will fit you perfectly. It will be custom made for you—washed, pressed, and ready for you to wear out into the world.

# # #

CHAPTER ELEVEN
PUTTING IT ALL TOGETHER

In the early part of the twentieth century, the pharmaceutical companies began to develop and promote their products in earnest. Many doctors became addicted to prescribing drugs provided by the pharmaceutical companies. Now, they have become totally dependent on each other.

Even though cancer is the second leading cause of death in the United States, the treatment for cancer hasn't changed very much in the last seventy years. The side effects of radiation (in use for over 100 years) and chemotherapy (in use since the 1940s), can be devastating. And, of course, they often don't work. So, why do people continue to go to doctors who torture them and destroy the quality of their lives? They do this because the collective ego has bought into the propaganda coming from the pharmaceutical companies and the medical community.

We all come and go. To most people, death seems like the ultimate betrayal, yet, death is part of life. Sometimes, ego will see death as preferable to change, but more often than not, it sees death as an intolerable loss, something to be avoided at all costs. This is a major reason you are willing to let your doctor use those barbaric procedures and nearly kill you.

Almost everyone who dies from cancer is receiving medical treatment. It looks like a valiant effort is being made to save your life, but, alas, the procedures are very dangerous and life-threatening. One of the side effects of radiation and chemotherapy is organ failure. Death from organ failure is not classified as dying from cancer. So the statistics can be misleading. In actuality, more people die every year from cancer than the numbers indicate.

A side effect of chemotherapy is extreme fatigue and you can't possibly earn a living while receiving treatment. All of this could be avoided if the medical community were to treat the actual *cause* of cancer, which is your mind. Of course, they would have to learn a new set of skills.

Life and death are really the same thing—two sides of the same coin. It is the ego that resists death. Death is a mystery. As you become more integrated, you become aware it is really just another experience in your on-going evolution. You are limited in your perception to what comes after death and that has a lot to do with ego's fear of it. Ego wants predictability and certainty. Of course, they don't exist. Those who are totally integrated do not fear death because they can see beyond this lifetime and are aware of their immortality. Yes, you are immortal, but you are not aware of it. You may not believe it, because the body you currently inhabit will turn to dust at some point. Just surrendering will often bring about a cure for your disease. If it doesn't, you will have many other lifetimes and opportunities to see your loved ones again.

Many of you will get cancer or other life-threatening diseases in the prime of life. The fact that you have been drawn to this book says a lot about you. You already have a connection to your Higher Nature, albeit modest, or you wouldn't be reading this book. You may think you have come to this information out of coincidence or desperation, but that's not entirely true. You may indeed be desperate, but that's not the sum total of why you have responded to this book. It's also a good indicator that you can survive your disease.

The idea that you are completely alone in this lifetime and not being guided and supported by the universe is completely false. It's the arrogance of ego trying to claim its authority over your life. Yield to everything that comes into your life; stop saying no to what you experience and you will find healing and peace. Surrendering is not just a passive step. It is the most dynamic stance you can take, because it enlists the assistance of your Higher Nature. It allows the wisdom of the universe to come to your aid, to solve problems, and heal. It is as simple as surrendering to the peace that is within you. Wisdom is right there, where you are right now, but it is obscured by your conditioning.

You are actually being lifted into a higher state of awareness as you read this book and begin to realize who you are. Maybe you don't completely understand what I am getting at, but rest assured, it is your Divine nature pointing you in a new direction. Some of you may think you don't need all of this spiritual stuff in order to heal, but why else would you be reading this? If you still feel that way, it is because your ego is digging in its heels. It is your choice. You can sell out to your ego, or not. The tools for healing are presented in this book. Many people go through life without giving any consideration to who they are; they are totally ego driven. The result of not connecting with your divinity is suffering and premature death. If ignoring who you are were a successful strategy, life on earth would look very different.

The travesty of believing you are your thoughts and your mind is destroying humanity. You are not the Little Self, but you keep on insisting it is your true identity. Look around. All of the destruction and devastation you see could not possibly be the result of your Higher Nature. It is the result of ignorance—ignoring who you are. The Little Self is ignorance personified. It is destructive, not creative. There is really only one Self and it can do no harm. Wisdom cannot create ignorance. Your Higher Nature is incapable of creating polarity. You ignore who you are at your own peril.

Knowing who you are doesn't in any way diminish your ability to function in the world, but the Little Self would like to have you think it does. Knowing who you are will enhance your life and the work you do. There will be an ease and flow to life that simply isn't there now. It will improve your relationships with your family and children, even if the children are already adults. Remember, the key to life is acceptance. When you accept what happens in life, you will receive more love. **Acceptance brings peace, awareness, and even enthusiasm into your life. Those qualities are the elixir of healing.**

"If only we could all just get along," some people say, but the outer world is simply a reflection of the chaos and inner conflict that everyone has stored in their unconscious mind. Healing the world begins with you. There is a connection between all individuals on the earth and everything you do affects the whole. A new paradigm of self responsibility and healing is being created here. You can accept it—or not. As you take responsibility for your own well-being, you are assisting everyone on the planet.

There is nothing for the Little Self in a society where we all get along. Ego is invested in conflict. Maybe you don't see yourself as a person who fights with others, but just look inside. You will find conflict and judgment. It strengthens ego's sense of identity. There is no such thing as an ego that is not in conflict with something; it needs struggle in order to survive. The Little Self is incapable of peace. As you gain more understanding of how the Little Self works, its influence on your life will diminish.   The norm for life on this planet so far has been denial of responsibility for what you experience. You can see where this has led humanity.

You are responsible for how you respond to what happens in your life. I have a client whose mother-in-law attacks her and is extremely judgmental of her. Julie is constantly planning a counter attack, an argument to combat the onslaught of negativity she knows she will hear. What I suggested she do when her mother-in-law launched an attack was to use the breath technique. It will immediately sever the negative energy coming from her mother-in-law. When I first suggested this to Julie, she didn't see how anything could prevent her mother-in-law from continuing to assault her. Everyone has reactive patterns in their unconscious mind. If you didn't have them stored in your unconscious, you wouldn't react to another's attack. Ego, of course, loves a good fight.

Using the breath technique clears the issues on both sides. Julie's reactive patterns were being reflected back to her by her mother-in-law. Up until I pointed that out to her, Julie was unaware (in denial) of those patterns. Once they were cleared, there wouldn't be any reason for her mother-in-law to attack her and she would find someone *else* to fight with. Her mother-in-law was actually helping Julie, by pointing out what she needed to clear.

Not long ago, I was confronted while giving a talk on the nature of life. The person proudly pointed out that he didn't believe there was anything beyond his five senses. That was the Little Self rising up on its hind legs, thumping its chest like an 800-pound gorilla claiming its territory. The content of the mind is ego's smorgasbord. It is what the ego feeds on, and of course, it doesn't want to go hungry. New information is needed for growth, expansion, and change. When you are open to new experiences, you begin to create the space for peace and wisdom.

There is a fundamental shift coming in the energies that support life on the earth; the change will raise awareness and make it easier to heal. The energy is predicted to arrive on December 21, 2012 and it will have a profound effect on the planet. There will be a convergence of events that started almost 13,000 years ago.

The precession of the equinoxes began with the creation of The Milky Way Galaxy. If you were to draw a straight line through the center of the earth along its axis, it would point to a particular constellation of stars, but as the earth spins and wobbles on its axis, it points to a different constellation, approximately every two thousand years. This is called the precession of the equinoxes. It completes the entire cycle in slightly less than 26,000 years. At the end of this cycle, the earth's axis will again point to the place where it began. It actually takes 25,920 years to complete the precession. At the mid-point of the cycle, on December 21, 2012, the earth's axis, moon, and sun will be in alignment with the center of the Milky Way Galaxy. The axis will begin pointing to the constellation of Aquarius. This will create a tidal wave of transformational energies which will need to be integrated. We are also moving from third chakra dominance, where power and control are the focus, to the heart chakra. Its qualities are love, compassion, forgiveness, and healing.

Somehow, the ancients knew about the precession of the equinoxes. It was written about in The Vedas more than 10,000 years ago, and by the Sumerians. The Sumerians are the oldest civilization we know of. The Vedas call it the Cycle of Yugas. The word yuga is a Sanskrit word that means a "period of time." They divided the cycle into six periods, or yugas. They also named each period: the descending cycle begins with Satya, Treta, Dwapara, and ends with Kali Yuga. Because it is the furthest point in the cycle, it has a descending and ascending aspect. The names on the ascending side are repeated, beginning with Kali,

Dwapara, Treta, and Satya. We have just moved out of Kali Yuga into Dwapara and are starting back to where we began, almost 13,000 years ago. Kali is the most difficult period we experience. Wars, polarity, emotional trauma, chaos, competition, power struggles, plagues, and disease dominate this period. Unknown to most, is that we are actually moving up a spiral, and though it looks like we are moving back to the starting point, we are actually moving to a higher place on the spiral. This means that even though we repeat the cycle, it will never be as difficult as it was in the past. The ancients say that in the beginning of the cycle, we were totally integrated, balanced, and very highly evolved, but as we move away from the starting point, we become disintegrated and lose sight of our true nature.

The ancient Mayan calendar ends on December 21, 2012, and because it doesn't extend beyond that date, some are predicting the end of the world, but I don't see that happening. I believe that it is really the dawn of a new era, an opportunity for transformation to a much higher state of awareness. This will be the beginning of the end of separation from your Higher Nature.

Past generations could not respond to what *The Course* says about disease, when it said "all disease is of the mind." It was ahead of its time. Self-awareness was simply not understood by most people, because the energy of the planet did not support it. Awareness and insight were believed to be qualities of the personality. Few knew that they were qualities of your Higher Nature. Oprah Winfrey, Deepak Chopra, Wayne Dyer, and others have started to create a new paradigm for millions of their viewers and readers. One of the qualities they emphasize is the importance of taking responsibility for your life. If you don't take responsibility for your own health and well-being, no one else will.

Almost eight million people die world-wide every year of cancer and as I pointed out in Chapter One, over

500,000 thousand die every year of cancer, in the U.S. They died because they believed they could turn their health over to an outside agent, namely the medical community. Turning your health over to someone else breaks the sacred contract you have with your Higher Nature.

You have been given autonomy by the universe, but you have forgotten this sacred contract exists. The agreement is you are never alone, or abandoned; you are always supported by the universe. But in order to reinstate that agreement, you have to stop identifying with the Little Self and begin integrating with the Big Self. You can do that by using the breath technique or by meditating. If you have faith and trust in the universe, it will support you.

Disease is a sign that you have lost sight of who you are. You have contracted your energies and have closed down, in order to protect yourself. Feelings, as you know, are one of the highest qualities that humans possess. Without being connected to your feeling nature, you will lose your connection to the healing force of the universe. Feeling is the bridge between you and your Higher Nature.

You know by now that whatever enters your unconscious mind becomes your reality. As an adult, you have a choice either to clear those negative patterns and reclaim your authority over life, or continue struggling and suffering.

Without a basic understanding of how life actually works, you will not be able to cope with disease or life. It was suggested earlier that you could easily clear unconscious patterns that create disease. Could it really be that simple, especially in light of the fact that medicine has adopted so many complex procedures? The answer is yes, but it takes a little skill and understanding, which is provided within this book. Many people have been brainwashed into thinking that complexity is important, but it is man, not God, who has introduced complexity into the process of healing.

Thus far, you have gained new insights into how disease is created and how to heal. If you have received a cancer diagnosis, I make the following recommendation. Before you acquiesce to your ego's version of healing, which always includes suffering and pain, go to the website www.cancertruth.org and read some of the articles posted there. If you take these ideas to your doctor, he will protest and cry foul. He may even start quacking like a duck! That is the 800-pound gorilla (ego) defending its turf. That said, many of you may still turn to traditional medicine for help; however, you now know a viable alternative is available.

# # #

ACTION STEPS FOR
HEALING AND PREVENTION OF DISEASE

A new healing paradigm is being created, where mind and self- awareness are the primary forces behind healing. The key to healing is in developing self-awareness. The primary tools for creating awareness are: meditation, the breath technique, self-inquiry, intention, and willingness to explore your unconscious mind. These tools will help enormously with the prevention of disease.

Because meditation is the first line of defense for prevention and is important to healing and releasing stress, a complete description of Vipassana meditation from Chapter One is included in these action steps:

"Respiration is an object of attention that is readily available to everyone, because we all breathe from the time of birth until the time of death. It is a universally accessible object of meditation. To begin, sit down, assume a comfortable, upright posture, and close your eyes. Turning from the outer world to the world within, you find that the most prominent activity is your own breathing. So, you give attention to this object, the breath entering and leaving the nostrils.

"The effort is not to control the breath, but instead to remain conscious of it as it naturally is: long or short, heavy or light, rough or subtle. For as long as possible one fixes the attention on the breath, without allowing any distractions to break the chain of awareness.

"As meditators we find out at once how difficult this is. As soon as we try to keep the mind fixed on respiration, we begin to worry about a pain in the legs. As soon as we try to suppress all distracting thoughts, a thousand things jump into the mind: memories, plans, hopes, fears. One of these catches our attention, and after some time we realize that we have forgotten completely about breathing. We begin again with renewed determination, and again after a short time, we realize that the mind has slipped away without our noticing."

Meditation connects you to the right side of your brain for intuition, creativity, wisdom, awareness, and your spiritual center.

Meditation quickens healing, lowers blood pressure, reduces stress, increases mental abilities, and strengthens the immune system.

Another excellent choice is Kundalini (yoga) meditation. One of my favorite teachers is Harijiwan Khalsa; you can find him on The Web. This form of meditation has the added benefit of clearing the chakras. Some other ways to release stress are yoga exercises, or Chi Gong, an ancient Chinese energy practice.

Look at what you are experiencing in your life. Your experiences are telling you what your beliefs are. No exceptions.

It is either "obstacle or "flow." Obstacles are negative feelings and thought forms that have solidified and become beliefs. Healing is there for you on the other side of those obstacles.

Use the breath technique to clear negative thought forms and beliefs. To begin: Close your eyes, breathe deeply, relax, and put all of your attention on your breathing. Breathe a little deeper than you would ordinarily. The breath technique will connect you to your Higher Nature for clearing, wisdom, healing, and solutions to problems. Use this process whenever you are feeling stress or simply need more clarity and direction.

In order to clear negative beliefs, you need to find and identify them. Disease occurs when you are in a contracted state; fear and negative thoughts contract your energies. Here are two approaches you can take: Make a list of limiting beliefs from what you experience, or, use the emotional discomfort you feel. Dive into the discomfort or negative beliefs and let the energy out of them.

Express your anger. Use a child's light-weight plastic baseball bat, throw a pillow on top of your bed, and visualize someone you are angry with. Then, beat the stuffing out of your pillow while screaming and cursing— "that S.O.B.!" or any other expletives that you use when you are angry. You can also scream into a pillow or a folded bath towel; they will muffle the sound.

Energy follows thought. Negative thoughts create low, slow frequencies, which encourage the growth of disease.

Negative thinking creates hopelessness and despair, so monitor your thoughts.

To stop negative thinking, visualize a stop sign and say—STOP, silently to yourself. If there are a lot of intense, negative thoughts, you may have to repeat the process a number of times.

Dive into the emotions or feelings that have created your malady. Once you find the pattern, just acknowledge and embrace it. Your awareness will clear the issue.

Self-awareness takes commitment and discipline. It facilitates healing and unlocks the gifts of your own uniqueness.

Another technique to help you strengthen your connection to your Higher Nature is to: Sit down, close your eyes, and put yourself in a light meditative state. Create a symbol for your Higher Nature. It can be any symbol: the sun, the moon, the Milky Way Galaxy, or anything else that feels right for you. Suspend your thoughts and intensely focus on your symbol. Do this daily; it will strengthen your connection and help you to discover who you are.

To merge with your Higher Nature: Pick a quiet spot, close your eyes, and go into a light meditative state. Simply ask the question, "Who Am I? Then, let go, surrender, and notice what's there before you start thinking again.

Give up judgment, especially right and wrong. They are the domain of ego; ego is trying to show that it is in control. When you judge something to be right or wrong, good or bad, you are hardening your position and strengthening your ego.

Surrender to your life experiences. Acceptance is the key to life and healing.

Look for grace in everything you experience, even the negative.

You are autonomous. Nothing outside of you has any influence on your life.

Your inner programs are reflected back to you by others. This is one of the hardest things for humans to understand, that their own inner landscape creates everything they experience.

You must maintain a positive **can-do** attitude in order to heal.

You will find it very difficult to heal your life, if at the same time you are replicating those old patterns and beliefs. Your stance has to be—**bring it on!** Stand your ground. Don't wimp out on yourself.

You have the power to create change, but your ego wants you to believe that you don't; it will try to distract you from this work, if it can.

# # #

PART II

PROSPERITY IN TOUGH TIMES

I

This book has not been written for the purpose of entertainment. It is a course on surviving life-threatening diseases and creating prosperity. The stakes could not be higher. When there is a life-threatening disease like cancer, it is almost always devastating to a person's finances. Because this is a course, I have broken one of the cardinal rules in writing. Namely, the one that says you should not repeat what you've already said. Since repetition is the only way most people learn, I feel justified in breaking that rule.

Because the cure for disease and poverty are so similar, you'll find that some of the ideas in Part I are repeated in Part II. If you find this offensive, you may want to skip this section of the book, however, there are some unique concepts in this material on prosperity that you won't find anywhere else. Of course, it's your choice to continue on—or not.

After beating the odds with cancer or some other life-threatening disease, you now have to cope with a difficult financial situation. You have used up all of your savings, spent the money in your 401K, and have gone deeply into debt. Even so, it is possible for you to restore your financial integrity.

The way back to prosperity is the same for everyone, no matter the cause. Indeed, these are tough times. Here in the United States and all around the world, people are struggling to survive. Formerly prosperous, well-run companies have closed their doors and laid off their employees. Everywhere you look, people are losing their jobs. Stock markets are threatened and governments across the world have gone deeply into debt, spending great sums of money to prop up their failing economies. Things are downright scary to say the very least. Perhaps as you read this, economic conditions are improving. They always do, but because of the cyclic nature of these events, this scenario will repeat itself. You will find yourself facing yet another test of your ability to survive in tough times.

Whether your financial situation is because of battling a disease, difficult economic times, or both, you are going to have to make some changes in order to survive and prosper. Until now, you have embraced the past, but the old ways simply aren't working anymore. It's time for you to create a new paradigm. You will discover, as you take on the new model being presented here, that fear and insecurity will disappear. All that will be left are abundance and prosperity.

As you integrate this new model and adopt what is being put forth, you will grow and prosper, even in tough times. It won't matter what is going on in the world around you. Creating a life of abundance and prosperity is everyone's goal, yet few attain it. Most of you have been taught that to become successful, you have to get a better education, make sacrifices, and work longer hours. In other words—join the rat race. If you just had more "stuff," a younger partner, a bigger house, a new sports car, then you would be satisfied—or so you think. It's easy to become lost in accumulating "things," yet no matter how much stuff you acquire, it will always seem that something is missing. If you are struggling to survive, then you are probably thinking,

"So what? Just show me the money!" Life can be hell on earth, when you can't pay your rent.

Our society places a lot of emphasis on being successful. Those who make it to the top in financial circles are idolized. CEO's and rich celebrities are paraded in front of us on the daily talk shows; the stories of the rich and powerful are captivating. It seems that the rich keep getting richer and the poor keep getting poorer. During political cycles, there is a constant debate on how to solve this issue. Well-meaning politicians try to come up with new solutions to this problem, yet nothing changes. The rich become richer and the poor keep sliding deeper into poverty.

One solution used by government is to take more of what the rich have and give it to the poor. Massive amounts of taxes are being collected by governments and are being redistributed, but it makes little difference, if any. This will never solve the problem. Every year, more people fall into poverty. Those who depend on government handouts and charity get locked into a downward spiral of dependency and poverty. Stop hoping for someone or something to bail you out. You are autonomous and unless you stop looking for help "outside" of yourself—nothing will change.

You are an unlimited being, with unlimited potential and creativity. You may be thinking if this is really true, then "Why am I not experiencing it?" What stops you from achieving your desires? What stands in your way? Is it your experience that no matter which way you turn, you are stopped dead in your tracks before you can build any real momentum?

Mortals cannot ordinarily see far enough or well enough into the future, to avoid mistakes. All wealthy people have experienced losses and most are constantly on guard, dreading the time when the pendulum swings in the opposite direction. Constant vigilance creates a lot of stress and feelings of insecurity. Stress can ruin your health and even kill you. It's not wealth that you want anyway. What you are really searching for are peace and fulfillment.

Most people are totally unaware of why they suffer and struggle to survive. You are poor and struggle because of your conditioning, beliefs, and because you don't know who you are. Notice, these are the same conditions that lead to disease. As you know, your conditioning and beliefs are being reflected back to you from others. It always looks like what you see in others has nothing to do with you, but the universe has provided this as a way for you to see your own beliefs and conditioning. Can this be changed? Absolutely! But it can't be without doing something about your conditioning and beliefs. What you see in others is like a radar beam showing you what lies ahead, unless you make changes and create a new model for your life. Nothing is as important to prosperity as becoming aware of how your conditioning and beliefs around money influence your life.

Your conditioning is tenacious and you will have to be disciplined in order to counteract it and create a new paradigm. You are not powerless. You can create your life any way you want it. You can actually have what you desire.

Those of you who integrate this information will never again have to worry about external forces and circumstances. Why? Because, security is an "inside" job. You will be secure because of what you have learned about how prosperity is created. A rich person who is totally wiped out is very likely to become wealthy again if they are aware that prosperity comes from within. When they know they are absolutely responsible for everything that happens to them, they realize it is possible to rebuild. When they are not self-responsible, they will fall into hopelessness and despair.

You can become habitually successful, though it will take a deep understanding of how prosperity is created. Many teachers emphasize a rather superficial and materialistic view of success. They don't understand how creation actually works, nor do they seem to realize that having a lot of stuff doesn't equate to fulfillment. We live in a very materialistic world where successful people are placed on a pedestal, especially by the media. It's easy to be influenced by them; they promote the idea that success is relative to how many things you acquire and how much money you have in the bank.

My own quest for understanding the nature of reality and how we actually create success came out of the pain and suffering of nearly two decades of financial successes and failures. Like many who suffer great losses, I began searching for the reasons behind them.

There are many teachers of success principles. You may have read books and taken classes on becoming successful and developing a millionaire mind, yet you continue to experience lack and limitation in your life. Why? Because most of those courses and books are focused on the "outcome," rather than on the "source" of your creativity and success—your Higher Nature/the Creative Self. It is like they are starting the race at the finish line. The Bible says, "Seek ye first the kingdom of heaven and all else will be given unto you."

Most of you have heard of the Law of Attraction. The majority of teachers will tell you that in order to create what you want, you must first make a list of your desires, set goals, create vision boards, visualize the outcome, think positive thoughts, and monitor your self-talk. They also tell you to pay attention to your feelings and to maintain an attitude of gratitude. If that were the entire process, all of their students would be fabulously successful. Yet, the majority of people who have taken classes and learned those techniques have not had a lot of consistent success. The key word here is "consistent." If your desire is simply to have a new red Corvette or some other "thing," then you may be able to create it by using those techniques. If you want to turn your life into a joyous creation of abundance and prosperity, making a list and doing those techniques will not help you very much to achieve it.

There are five laws that greatly affect your ability to create your desires. The only one you are likely to hear about is the Law of Attraction, and while it is important, it is just one of the five laws critical to your success. The laws being talked about here are always working for you, but your conditioning and beliefs diminish their power. You can reclaim their original strength and enhance their effectiveness.

The Law of Attraction

The following information on the Law of Attraction comes from *The Teaching of the Inner Christ,* by Ann Meyer Makeever. She claims this material was given to her in the early 1960s by an ancient Being, called Babaji. He appeared in her living room and gave her the entire course.

"The Law of Attraction is the drawing force which centralizes ideas into purpose and purposeful activity. It is the cohesive quality of being the pull which holds Being together. This law operates on the level of spirit and is always attracting good to us and is ever seeking goodness for all of life. On the mental level, it operates by our thoughts and beliefs, attracting their likeness into our experience. On the physical level, this law operates as the pull of gravity. Through the Law of Attraction, similar vibrations come together and similar purposes join themselves into activities of greater power. On the human level, this law draws together groups and persons of similar intent. Through this law, personal relationships are formed according to the choice and purposes of those involved. Families are created which weave themselves together in varying relationships through many incarnations. This very law is the drawing force which combines the words of the sentences in this book and the sentences into chapters or clusters of ideas. Thus the Law of Attraction simplifies the complexities of Being and allows them to be better understood and experienced.

"This law can be called upon to bring into our lives persons or experiences we desire, or eliminate persons or experiences which do not belong in our lives at the present time. The opposite of attraction is repulsion. Unlike purposes, intents tend to repel one another. That which is not in harmony with our purpose are, by this law, repelled from us and leave our experience."

The Law of Correspondence

The Law of Correspondence is as important as the Law of Attraction. It is also called the Law of Equivalents. It says that for every question there is an answer, and for every problem there is a solution. When you are looking for answers to questions, or solutions to problems, you can meditate on the Law of Correspondence. The answers may not always come in your meditations, but they will come to you in one way or another. They may show up in your thoughts, your dreams, intuitively, or as impressions and feelings. If you don't already know how to meditate, it's about time you learned.

The Law of Correspondence says that when you hold a belief or an idea in your mind, you will attract corresponding beliefs and ideas that will come together and create an experience. It also says that thoughts will tend to attract their likeness. That's the reason you need to monitor your thoughts. According to this law, what you see in others and judge, you will experience within yourself.

The Law of Abundance

The Law of Abundance is also called the Law of Multiplication. It is where God said to go forth and multiply. The Law of Abundance is governed by acceptance. The inability to accept what you desire comes from beliefs in your unconscious mind. Appreciation and gratitude are also an aspect of the Law of Abundance. They are important and assist you with being able to receive what you desire. Gratitude and appreciation create openness and receptivity.

One of the keys to obtaining what you desire lies in your willingness to accept love. It is very likely that if you are experiencing financial difficulties, you are also having difficulty accepting love. Often, the belief that is keeping you from love is the same one that creates lack and limitation. Many of you have a belief that you don't deserve love.

If you cannot let love in, then prosperity and abundance will elude you. Not being able to accept love is the result of the fear created by love being conditional as a child. Fear limits your ability to accept abundance and love. Fear and love are opposites. Love is the creative force; fear creates more fear, lack, and limitation.

Actually, everything that comes to you from the Creative Self is to help you create prosperity and abundance. This is the natural state of the universe. Everything you receive from your Higher Nature/the Creative Self will assist you. There is only well-being coming to you, but you cannot accept it because of your conditioning and beliefs.

Most teachers of prosperity and abundance principles believe that thought is how you create and manifest in your life, but they are only partially correct. Belief is far more powerful than thought. A powerfully charged negative belief is unlikely to be overcome by thought alone. If you were to stop thinking all together and live entirely in the moment, you would create the most abundant life imaginable. Thought is often in conflict with what the Creative Self is trying to create for you.

Eckhart Tolle, author of *A New Earth,* says it like this: "If the thought of lack—whether it be money, recognition, or love—has become part of who you think you are, you will always experience lack. The fact is: Whatever you think the world is withholding from you, you are withholding from the world. You are withholding it because deep down you think you are small and that you have nothing to give.

"Whatever you think people are withholding from you—praise, appreciation, assistance, loving care, and so on—give it to them. If you don't have it, just act as if you had it, and it will come. Then, soon after you start giving, you will start receiving. You cannot receive what you don't give. Outflow determines inflow. Whatever you think the world is withholding from you, you already have, but unless you allow it to flow out, you won't even know that you have it. The law that outflow determines inflow is expressed by Jesus in this powerful image: 'Give and it will be given to you.'

"The source of all abundance is not outside you. It is part of who you are. However, start by acknowledging and recognizing abundance without. The acknowledgment of the abundance that is all around you awakens the dormant abundance within. Then let it flow out. When you smile at a stranger, there is already a minute outflow of energy. You become a giver. Ask yourself often: 'What can I give here, how can I be of service to this person, this situation?' Abundance comes only to those who already have it. Both abundance and scarcity are inner states that manifest as your reality."

The Law of Expansion

This law says, that "what you put your attention on, increases." All things have the desire to grow and expand. The universe is expanding. Concepts, ideas, and thoughts held over time, tend to grow and expand.

Life always seeks growth. Each of us wants to enhance our abilities and skills; you especially want to express yourself. When not growing, learning, and having new experiences, you feel frustrated and limited. In order to grow and evolve, you must be willing to change; this is one of the hardest things for humans to do. Everyone desires growth and expansion, yet you resist and adhere to the old ways of doing things.

The Law of Mind

The most important law of the five is the Law of Mind. This law says "As you believe, so shall you receive." The Bible says, "It is done unto you according to your belief." Everything you experience is subject to this law. There are no exceptions. The Law of Mind cannot be violated. None of the laws being talked about are effective by themselves. They all work in concert and are subject to the Law of Mind.

Many teachers are unaware of this law. As a result, they lead their students to believe they can create their desires without doing anything about their negative beliefs. Beliefs are energetic patterns in your field and once a pattern is created, it will dominate your experience from that point on, or until the energy is released from it. Patterns and beliefs become magnetic and attract their own likeness.

One of the things you want to watch out for is making your suffering and losses "real." By focusing on and judging them, you are empowering failure. Judgment amplifies negative patterns by adding energy to them. Making your failures real will strengthen your beliefs in lack and limitation and will create even more of it. Remember— the Law of Expansion states that "What you put your attention on grows and expands."

The back and forth swing of the pendulum creates the feeling of insecurity that most people have—you either become overly optimistic or overly pessimistic. All of this can be avoided. When you stop giving your power to what you are trying to create, and focus on the real source of your personal power, the Creative Self, you will begin to live life as a master creator and you will be much less affected by the fickle nature of duality. Whatever setbacks come your way will be minimized and quickly overcome.

If you take my advice, you will form an intimate connection with the Creative Self. How will you know when you have formed that connection? It is simply a feeling that has no defining characteristics. It's a sense of well-being, a knowing that you are that magnificent Being and creative force. Why is this important to prosperity and abundance? Because, if you are able to grasp this concept, you will begin to give up believing that your limitations are "real." The strength of your connection to the Creative Self determines how successful you will be. All things finite are illusion. This simple act of making the "unreal," "real," is the major reason it's so easy to get caught in a downward spiral that ends in despair and hopelessness. There is no failure—just experience. Judgment always energizes whatever is being judged.

Once you have connected to the Creative Self, it is entirely possible that you will never have to deal with limited finances ever again. If you do not avoid some loss, the pendulum will always swing the other way. There is always an "up" cycle and if you don't make your losses real, you will pull out of it quickly. It will be just another bump along your road to prosperity.

The only real security you have comes directly from the Creative Self, because ego and personality are not in the least bit creative. They create absolutely nothing of value. They simply get in the way of the creative process.

Many of you dwell on your history, continuously talking about how difficult life was as a child and how it has followed you into adulthood. You see yourself as a victim. You cannot change the past by reliving your story over and over; you are actually projecting your past into the future. You cannot regain your personal, creative power while at the same time you are complaining and blaming others for what you have experienced. Blame makes you powerless.

Some of you have taken classes on becoming successful, yet you have not succeeded. Most teachers believe that creation begins with thought. The actual creative equation looks like this:

The Creative Self + Mind + Belief + Thought = Creation

As you can see, thought is indeed a part of the equation, but it really is the least important part. What you need to know is that the creative equation begins with the Creative Self and that it is not in any way affected by duality or the relative world we live in. Thoughts give direction to beliefs. They are not the entire process—only a small part of it.

The path to a more satisfying life requires two things: A deep connection to the Creative Self, so that it can speak to you of a grander purpose, and clearing negative beliefs keeping you from becoming prosperous. Something more fulfilling is available to anyone who is willing to do these two things.

Remember—you are the creator of your life. You are not at the mercy of it. You are creating your life moment-to-moment—right now. Nothing exists until the Creative Self manifests it. You are creating everything, including the money in your bank account.

The Creative Self does not experience limitation; it is totally creative. The life you are experiencing is an "illusion." It exists only as a reflection of the Creative Self and your mind. If the Creative Self wants to create a lot of money in your bank account, all it has to do is select a template in your hologram that has a lot of money in it. Mind then energizes it and it will show up as a deposit in your bank account. And, the good news is—you can spend it in any way you want. However, the Creative Self may not see that as your best option. Instead, it may choose to create a new job or career for you. It may be similar to what you are doing now or it may be something entirely new and different. But, it will be fulfilling.

When you actually get this—that you are autonomous and that you are One with the most creative force in the universe, you will be successful no matter what is going on around you. No matter how tough times are for others, you will be successful.

Manifesting is about being "in the flow" with the Creative Self, allowing it to guide and direct your life. At times, this will mean acquiring more "things," but it will always mean whatever is most rewarding and fulfilling at that time. As you become more connected to the Creative Self, what you find fulfilling, will change. It simply cannot remain the same. As you move through life reconnecting with it and clearing those old failure patterns, everything will change. A great deal of fulfillment is derived by simply discovering your true nature.

Don't look now, but there's an 800-pound gorilla standing in the middle of your kitchen! Like with all ferocious beasts, it's a little hard to know how to approach it. Overlooking and not confronting a gorilla in your kitchen might seem impossible, but most people would accommodate the beast, rather than engage it. This makes sense, doesn't it? After all, who would choose to confront such a Goliath? If you haven't figured it out already, the gorilla is your ego. Comparing your ego to an 800-pound gorilla may seem a bit far-fetched, but it's not. They share similar qualities. They are powerful, tenacious, and aggressive when it comes to defending their turf. And, whether you know it or not, you are pitted against that mighty hulk. It will never give up its territory without a fight.

Your ego is the part of you that identifies with mind, conditioning, beliefs, and thought. Conditioning and beliefs are the biggest hurdles to creating the prosperity and abundance you desire. The paradox is that your ego wants you to be successful, but it resists change.

Almost everything you desire is the result of ego's insecurity. Trust has been replaced by fear. The Limited Self (ego) demands that its needs be filled, so that it can be at peace and feel secure. This is a real Catch 22: the Limited Self demands that its desires be accommodated, but it can never be fulfilled by acquiring more "stuff." The gorilla may seem powerful, but because ego is fear-based, it has no real power—yet, it seems to.

Not far from my home, there is a Safeway store. Often there are homeless people standing on the street corner selling a newspaper called *Real Change*. It is published by a charity organization for the poor and the homeless to sell for only a dollar. Many people walk right past them without buying a paper. It's rare that I pass one of them without stopping and purchasing a copy, but when I do, I don't get very far before I turn around and go back to buy one. Why? Because the thought of not having enough money to share contracts your energy and blocks the flow of money to you. You cannot play the game of life this way and win it. The game can't be won when it's built on a foundation of scarcity and limitation. The act of giving opens your heart and places you in a receptive state. It feels good to give, and feeling good opens you to the flow of life and abundance. Generosity begets generosity.

You see yourself as limited, simply because your parents, schools, churches, and other institutions have coerced you into going along with what they believed: "Don't be a rebel and don't be different." "Simply blend in, and most importantly, don't make waves." After all, you are just another nameless face in the crowd who is trying to survive a perilous life.

You are not who you think you are. You are much more than your conditioning. You are the unlimited power of creation, masquerading as a human. You are not powerless to change, but you may believe that you are. You will find it very difficult to achieve prosperity, if at the same time you are replicating those old patterns of scarcity and limitation.

The patterns and beliefs in your unconscious mind were created by you, perhaps unconsciously, but never the less at your request. The Creative Self winked at you when you chose them, knowing all the while they weren't real—that they were only a temporary diversion from the truth. It takes tremendous energy to hang onto those old, limiting patterns. Indeed, you could be using that same energy to create the life you desire. The patterns you took on as a child helped you survive your childhood, but they no longer serve you. You can crack the shell that protects them and let the energy out of them. Once they are exposed to self-awareness, they will no longer affect your life. They will be replaced by patterns that will support your new paradigm. Clearing patterns is like letting the air out of a tire. Once the energy is released, the pattern ceases to move forward and distort your life.

The following is the same process used in Chapter Six for clearing beliefs around disease, but as you can see, the focus is now on beliefs around money. There are two approaches you can take at this point. You can make a list of limiting patterns from what you experience. Like—"I never have enough money to pay my bills." Or, you can use the emotional discomfort you feel to identify what needs to be cleared. It's OK to do both.

Take a good look at your life and ask yourself, "What financial limitations do I currently experience?" Money is certainly a big issue for most. Often, there will be a cluster of patterns around money. "Money is hard to come by." "I am always broke." "Money slips through my fingers." "Money is evil." "Money doesn't grow on trees," or, "People with money are greedy and stingy." A belief such as "I never have enough money," will often be supported by beliefs around not being deserving: "I don't deserve to have money, or, "I don't deserve to have what I want." These are some other beliefs that may be on your list: "I never get what I want," "I am powerless to change," "Nothing ever works out," My efforts never pay off," "I am unworthy, and "I don't deserve love." You may find many variations around the same belief.

Once you have discovered a belief or an emotional pattern that you want to clear, dive into it and feel it as deeply as you can. Stay with the feeling and immerse yourself in it. It may begin to intensify. Stay with the intensity as best you can. You will never get more than you can handle. When you feel like the intensity has peaked, ask the Creative Self to transmute it or to release the energy from the pattern.

How will you know if you are making progress? As you clear the unconscious mind of unwanted debris and conditioning that holds you back, your connection to your Higher Nature/the Creative Self will be strengthened and change will begin to occur.

Prosperity will begin to show up and you will find your life changing in ways you are not accustomed to. Change will accelerate, as you become more self-aware. What is required is that you take the time to do the simple techniques offered in this material.

If you have spent your life focused on the "outer" world, you will need to become more inwardly directed. After all, you are creating a new paradigm for your life, where commitment to change is your greatest ally.

# # #

II

Somewhere in our history, perhaps even today in remote places of the world, there are those who can shape shift. There are ancient traditions being taught today called The Siddhis, where people learn to levitate, disappear, and instantly create anything they desire. Magicians and illusionists appear to be shape shifting right before our eyes.

Stories abound the world over about a large, hairy being that stands on two legs and walks through the forest. In Washington State, where I live, it's called Big Foot. It is known as the Indomitable Snowman, or the Yeti, in The Himalayas. Is this creature actually shape shifting or is it miraculously moving between different dimensions? Or, is it just a myth? Shape shifting in the way it is being used here, simply means morphing into your unlimited nature. For most, this is a shift so monumental, that it could be called shape shifting.

You already know that your power base is the Creative Self. Certainly, most of you do not have the connection to the Creative Self that you would like to have. Restoring the connection to your own creative power is likely very enticing and exciting for you. It's much like meeting an old friend that you grew up with and haven't seen for many years. For reasons we have talked about, you turned away as a child, from who you really are, into a person bound by ego, fear, and limitation. Now, you are becoming aware of the possibility of shifting back into the unlimited version of yourself.

As you read this, you may be wondering if it is worth the time and effort required to revert back to your unlimited nature? After all, you have a job, a family, your favorite TV show, house cleaning and shopping to do, a partner, and some classes you want to attend at the nearby community college. And, don't forget the books you haven't finished, waiting for you on the nightstand next to your bed. There just isn't enough time in the day to work something new into your cluttered schedule. All of this may seem like it's true—but, it's not. What's really going on is the part of you that resists change is creating a strategy to keep you limited. Morphing back into the Unlimited Self that you were when you were born is just too scary for the ego to think about. It's really just a tradeoff. It's a choice, albeit one that comes with a goodly amount of resistance. The choice is to either live as a powerful creative force, or to live your life by default and limitation.

The one creature we all know of that can shape shift and morph into a new form, is the caterpillar. It instinctively spins a cocoon and falls asleep; it doesn't have to deal with resistance and belief systems. Some morph into beautiful Monarch butterflies and have the tenacity to migrate thousands of miles every year.

How hard is it to become a shape shifter? Not as difficult as it may seem. As you know, these are tough times and this implies you are going to have to learn some new skills in order to prosper: Learn to meditate, use the breath technique, or sit for a few minutes every day with your eyes closed and do self-inquiry. Remember—self-inquiry begins with the question "Who am I?" Spend a few minutes each day clearing patterns. Abundance just is. Limitation and scarcity are not real; they are part of the illusion. As you make the shift inward, you will begin to morph back into the powerful creative force that is your natural state.

You are limited in your ability to shape shift because you are identified with the Limited Self. Think about that for a moment. At this stage of your understanding, you will probably see yourself as limited. That is what you have been taught to believe is true. Yet, all of the major religions and spiritual teachings tell us something else. Even Christianity and the Bible say you are created in the image of God; Christianity is quiet about the part that says God and you are "One." It is self-serving for religions to keep quiet about who you are.

If you attend one of Tony Robbins' classes, or The Millionaire Mind Workshops taught by T. Harv Eker, you will come out feeling like you are king of the world—that you can create a life of prosperity and abundance, with ease. Their presentations are impeccable; they know exactly how to motivate you. Many people who have worked with them claim they have achieved success. However, I have never met anyone who has experienced lasting success from any of those workshops. If you were to monitor their progress, you would see that it tends to diminish, as time passes. The reason for this is that they believe you can achieve success without doing the "inner" work. Even so, many continue to attend those workshops, still hoping to achieve their desires. Obviously, there are different strokes for different folks. Taking those classes may satisfy you for the short term, but sooner or later, you will come to the conclusion that you sincerely want to shift into something more lasting and fulfilling.

In the past, shape shifting was part of black magic traditions. It was used to gain personal power and control over others. The principle power behind shape shifting is the awareness that everything is illusion. Let's face it. If you have the power to create the illusion of being human, you also have the ability to shape your own personal illusion in any way you want it. Of course, you would first have to agree that what you are experiencing is illusion. You may be asking, "What's the proof?" " How do I know my life is really an illusion?" If, by that, you mean "scientific" proof that it's an illusion, just look to quantum physics. The founders of quantum physics were David Bohm, Niels Bohr, Werner Heinsenberg, and Dr. Albert Einstein. They all believed that life is really an illusion. Most, if not all of the modern quantum physicists agree. According to quantum physics, "The observer creates the observed" is a statement of fact.

Quantum physics makes it very clear that we are creating life moment-to-moment, as we observe it. No doubt, life seems real to you. And, whether you believe it is real or not, just by doing the simple things being suggested here, you will experience your own shift and begin to restore financial security.

Have you noticed that the media does not emphasize personal power? Maybe once a week, you'll find something on TV that is empowering, but you can be assured it will be shown very late at night or very early in the morning, during time slots when few are watching. An exception to this is Oprah, and occasionally, Larry King.

Both Larry King and Oprah had the teachers of *The Secret* on twice. *The Secret* is a DVD on the Law of Attraction. People thought it was very helpful. More than one million DVDs were sold within the first six months of production. When *The Secret* was introduced to the public, it wasn't long before mainstream media began to ridicule and try to suck the life out it. The media organizations didn't like their own influence being diminished by something as simple as the Law of Attraction.

The Law of Attraction says you can have anything you desire. "That's not possible," cried the media, so they found a psychiatrist and a behavioral scientist to criticize *The*

Secret. Those individuals just happened to be funded by a major university and the government. Keeping you powerless and dependent is the goal of government and most religions. Of course, the government wants you to believe you are powerful and don't need them. Oh, *sure* they do!

You are a "master creator" and are responsible for creating the good and the bad that you experience. The power you have within is incredible! Once you understand and truly believe this, you will be able to shape your reality "at will." The chair you are sitting in, the light you have turned on in order to read this information, and the book itself, have been created by you in the moment. You have a job, a car, a home, kids, and money in the bank—too little, perhaps, but nevertheless, you do have a bank account. These things don't actually exist except in your mind and imagination. You have projected those events into your hologram and have declared them "real." Once you get this at a very deep level, you will begin to shape your life in unimaginable ways. Nothing is concrete. Nothing is cast in stone. Everything is fluid and mutable. It looks to you like everything is subject to time. You need to be patient and things will work out, or so you hope. Look—if you are creating this life moment-to-moment, how much time can it really take to accomplish anything? Your sanity demands that there is some continuity, but it isn't really necessary.

According to quantum physics, you exist in a field of infinite potential. The Creative Self creates that field to play and create form—a sandy beach for it to create its version of sand art. You have seen how quickly a sand castle can be washed away by the ocean tide.

Think about this for a minute or two. All things, including this book, are really just patterns in your hologram that you perceive as real, solid, and concrete. If you look at anything that seems solid, through a powerful electron microscope, you will see that it is mostly empty space with atoms swirling about. According to quantum physics, those atoms are not even objects or things. Nothing is as it seems. Why? Because it's all illusion being created by you, to convince yourself that it's real, so that you can play the limitation game and have the experience of being human. It's no coincidence that movies like *Star Trek* and *The Matrix* are so popular. They actually show you how the illusion really works. The Holodeck on *Star Trek* is a good example of how your hologram actually works.

Power comes from truth and awareness. You can create whatever you desire. Those who have cleared their unconscious mind of limiting beliefs will gain enormous powers to create whatever they desire. However, there is a Catch-22 here. Those who become "clear" tend to desire less and are content to live a simple life. If you were to travel to India and visit some of the Indian saints living today in Southern India, you would find that they live a simple life and with very few of the things that most of us think we need in order to be comfortable. This is in spite of the fact that they can manifest anything they desire. What's their secret? It's a deep, abiding connection with the Creative Self. You have the same potential. You may never be as powerful as those Indian saints are, but you can be a lot more powerful than you presently are. We all live with some limitation, no matter what we have achieved, but, even that is self-imposed. There are no special souls. No one has any greater claim to potential than another. The creative process is the same for everyone.

Everyone is actually seeking peace. Abundance and prosperity are just metaphors for what you are really seeking. Few people find deep inner peace, but as you become more integrated, you will begin to experience it.

You could have peace, yet have nothing at all, or you could possess all of the things you could possibly desire—a mansion, a new sports car, or perhaps several sport cars (one for every day of the week), and a bank account with tons of money in it. You could have all of those things, yet not have peace.

A mansion and a sports car are just more ego stuff. It's so the ego can feel more powerful and secure. Don't get me wrong. I am not saying you should not have things. You deserve to have a comfortable home to live in, a nice car, a loving partner, or whatever else makes this lifetime rewarding.

The Limited Self (ego) is just pretending to be powerful. There is only one CEO and that is the Creative Self. That is where you want to put your focus; keep it there as much as you can. When you feel stressed and confused, use the breath technique. The Creative Self of course, is creative, but there is a peculiar catch to its creative ability. It is subjective, or passive. That is why the equation exists. Mind is where inspired action takes place, where desire is energized.

The definition of insanity is to keep doing the same thing over and over, expecting a different result. You keep hoping that somehow circumstances will change, but simply desiring change will not actually create it. You are on autopilot with those old, limiting patterns and it is insanity to think your life will change without doing the inner work.

In quantum physics there is the uncertainty principle put forth by Werner Heisenberg, one of the founders of quantum physics. He says that what is created is affected by choice. Unconsciously, you are choosing to create what you don't want. Observe what you encounter moment-by-moment and day-to-day. Look at what keeps showing up in your life. Those experiences are projections of patterns that have been energized in your mind. Lucky or smart are those who habitually ask themselves where their experiences come from and then stop to examine the patterns and clear them.

We have discussed the five laws that determine what you create and manifest. You could not experience life as you know it without the Law of Attraction and the other laws. They are always working for you, to create what you desire. A belief can come and go in a moment of time, but the laws are constant. You could probably deconstruct them if you wanted to, but for obvious reasons, it's not recommended.

There are two additional laws that impact your life and affect your ability to create what you desire: The Law of Compensation (also called the Law of Reciprocity) and The Law of Gender.

The Law of Compensation

The Law of Compensation says, "When you give your energy away, no matter what the form, it will always come back to you." It's like dipping a bucket of water from the ocean. It is quickly replaced and balance is restored. Nature abhors a vacuum and will always fill it. Jesus said, 'Give and you shall receive." That is why "generosity" is an important weapon in your prosperity arsenal.

The Law of Gender

The Law of Gender says, "Everything in its own time." In other words, everything has a gestation period. Let go of your need to have immediate results. Ego wants instant gratification, but the universe proceeds according to its own schedule—not yours. Earlier, I said that there is no reason you can't manifest what you want immediately, yet, this law says that everything has a gestation period. It's another paradox that cannot be easily explained.

As you clear your limiting patterns, you may not see progress as quickly as you want. It could take a month or more, but just be patient and stay the course. A monumental shift is being birthed and the universe may want you to have all of your ducks in a row before the changes occur.

Action Steps for
Creating Prosperity

Wait until you feel inspired to act. As you evolve, you will become more aware of what the Creative Self is directing you to do. Don't become proactive in this regard. Wait for inspiration and then act. It's easy to fall into the proactive mode. You may think you are being inspired when it's only your ego creating thoughts of grandiosity—those thoughts are always ego. You will know right away if something is coming from the Creative Self, because it will feel right and flow effortlessly.

It is out of inspiration that this book came about. One morning, just before I was totally awake, I had one of those big A-HA moments! I realized that the power mind plays in healing would be an excellent subject to write about.

Set your intention to make a dramatic change and to turn your life around.

Write out your financial goals. This one is tricky. Write out your goals only if you feel compelled to do so and then let go of them. Don't do this more than once. Your ego loves to create mind games by creating lists and making elaborate plans for the future. Those games will slow your progress and are likely to distort the message coming to you from the Creative Self. If you write them down more than once, you are creating a subtle message that you have failed to get what you want. It will reinforce your belief in failure.

Express appreciation when paying bills. Do not go into negative self-talk and judgment about your bills. You are the only one in your hologram, so you are actually paying yourself. Dive in and clear the belief, "I never have enough money to pay my bills." You received something by creating these bills. Show appreciation for what you have received. The words you use to express appreciation don't matter. It is the feeling that counts. You can't fake it. You have to actually feel it. You need to express appreciation for the money you receive—pay check, dividends, royalties, etc. If you feel like it's impossible to express appreciation, then stay neutral and away from negative, judgmental thoughts and feelings.

Set aside a few minutes each day, to explore who you are and build your power base. You can use the breath technique or the question "Who Am I?"

Make a strong, determined commitment to do the "inner" work. Commitment is the antidote to ego's resistance.

Ask the Creative Self to show you what your next step should be. Let go of your agenda and preconceived ideas of what your life should look like. In one way or another, the answer will come to you. It may come in a dream, while day dreaming, in a moment of clarity, or as a feeling. It may also come in your thoughts.

Monitor your thoughts, particularly if you have a lot of negative self-talk. Let go of your "stories." Stories will reinforce those negative patterns.

As you deepen your connection with the Creative Self, you will begin to clear those negative thought forms and patterns. A lot of negative patterns will clear as you become more aware of who you are.

Observe your resistance. You will have resistance. Acknowledge and embrace it. Do not confront it; that will only make it stronger. As you acknowledge and embrace your resistance, it will diminish.

Dive into those negative patterns and let the energy out of them! Set some time aside every day to work on clearing. You may be casual about the other steps, but if you really want to turn your life around and prosper, clearing those limiting obstacles is critical.

Stay focused. Remember—you will always get more of what you put your attention on.

Bring it on! Develop a **bring-it-on** attitude when it comes to finding and clearing those old, negative patterns. Actually, tell the Creative Self to bring them into your awareness.

Don't give up. Napoleon Hill, the author of *Think and Grow Rich,"* says that "Persistence is to men as carbon is to steel." Carbon makes steel strong.

Form a support group by getting together with like-minded people. This is an optional step. You may find strength in sharing your experiences and achievements with others. Stay away from people who don't support what you are doing. Your ego may bring "nay sayers" into your life to test your resolve. Stand your ground. You will be rewarded.

Connect with the Creative Self throughout your day.

Watch out for distractions. One way your ego resists is to distract you from your goals. You may forget to do the process or to take a few minutes out of your day to connect with the Creative Self. It's the Limited Self trying to distract you. Forgetfulness is always ego.

Acknowledge yourself for what you are experiencing and the courage it takes to change. Feel the fear and do it anyway!

As you start clearing your old, suppressed patterns, emotions or fear may arise. Don't quit. Just dive into them and ask the Creative Self to clear that fear.

As you take on the energy of the Creative Self, you will find yourself being guided through life without ever stepping on a land mine. Your life will begin to flow. Prosperity, abundance, and health will show up in your life in glorious and unexpected ways!

THE END

Epilogue

As you may know, my healing work began many years ago when I developed a system for clearing emotional issues. One of the lessons I learned since creating that process is that if you were to completely clear all emotional issues, fear, and anger, any and all of your disease(s) would disappear.

The system I created for clearing was specifically designed to clear suppressed emotions and feelings. I wasn't aware at the time that suppressed emotional issues cause disease. As I proceeded to work with clients, I discovered that many couldn't cope with their deeply suppressed emotions and feelings no matter how sincere they were about healing.

I developed a lot of skill at guiding them gently through their emotions and feelings. Emotions and feelings are really the same and can be used interchangeably. However, often when my clients got to their core issues--there are usually more than one--they just could not face the music, so to speak, and would not go deep enough to clear them, especially when there was emotional, physical, or sexual abuse involved. The most eager to heal would refuse to explore their feelings, and then many of them would quit working with me and stopped clearing altogether. Often I am my own guinea pig, as I experiment with developing new skills and abilities. I do my own exploration to determine what works and what doesn't.

A friend sent me some hypnosis CDs for sleep and weight loss. I was having some trouble sleeping at the time. The hypnotist said that all hypnosis is self-hypnosis. I took this literally, and after practicing for a few days, learned to hypnotize myself. The most important thing I learned as a result of participating in that process is that the subconscious mind will respond to your intention to open and explore it.

You can clear beliefs and conditioning at very deep levels when you open the subconscious mind. I began experimenting on myself. Every day while riding the bus to work at my part-time job, I practiced clearing my subconscious mind of conditioning and negative beliefs. The results were quite pleasing. My life began to flow more effortlessly and I became more prosperous. You can direct your intention to open your subconscious mind and enhance and deepen the effect of the clearing process. This can be very effective for healing and clearing beliefs that limit you financially.

The process I use to clear beliefs and conditioning is described in chapter six.

Now I had two powerful techniques to assist clients with clearing and healing: deep emotional healing and clearing negative beliefs from the subconscious mind.

I thought it couldn't get better than this, but it did.

One day while surfing You Tube, I came across some interesting information on healing. Some of it seemed a little esoteric, but that had not stopped me in the past and it didn't this time either. There was a video with testimonials about Braco, a well-known healer in Eastern Europe, who has worked with thousands of people.

The same day I saw an interview with Oprah and John of God, who is a healer living in a small village in

Brazil. Thousands of people go to see him every year for healing. There are reports of miraculous healings with both of these men. But no matter how good a healer is, some people who go to them will not be cured. The reason for this is that all disease has something to teach; there is a lesson to be learned from it. Until you know what that is you may not be able to heal, but once you understand why you have the disease you will be able to resolve it.

A number of years ago, a friend and I attended a workshop with Braco in Seattle, Washington. Suddenly my friend said, "Why don't you do what he is doing?" In other words, facilitate group healings. I thought to myself, his motivation in saying that may not be completely altruistic, since this auditorium is filled with people who had paid to attend the seminar. Yet he also realized there was a need and believed I had the skills necessary to do similar work. Little did I know at the time that not long after that comment, I would start working with groups of people who wanted to heal.

All healing occurs when the genes change their mind. They may not actually think, but they are intelligent. Genes respond to the environment they are in. In other words, they respond to the quality of energy they receive. When energy is transmitted to a person who has an emotional issue or a disease, the underlying emotional energy pattern breaks up. The genetic blueprint then changes to something more favorable. But it doesn't always have to be a disease. A woman whose neck was out alignment called me and said she needed a chiropractic adjustment but that most adjustments made her neck worse. She wanted to try something different. We simply did some energy work on her neck and after two sessions, her neck was completely back in alignment.

I worked solely via telephone with her. You may wonder how that works. In quantum physics, they say there is no time or space--they are an illusion; this has certainly been my experience. I have worked with hundreds of people all over the world by phone and had amazing results.

Up to that point, my efforts had been predominately focused on helping individuals clear emotional issues. Of course I had worked with people who had physical challenges, but they were not in the majority. When my friend made the comment to me about working with groups, I wondered if I was capable of transmitting enough energy to affect hundreds of people at the same time.

After attending the workshop with Braco, I remembered a book I had on one of my bookshelves, with a technique for creating a sphere of energy in the heart center and then transmitting it to people who desire healing. I had followed this author's work for years and had no reason to disbelieve what he was saying, so I worked diligently almost every day for over four months to build that reservoir of energy he described in his book. I began to practice on friends and then on a few select clients, and it indeed worked. People began experiencing healing where they were unable to before.

The energies I work with are conscious and extremely intelligent. They impact the atomic structure of the genes. They also clear the underlying beliefs and conditioning that cause disease.

I have spent a lot of time with many powerful healers. Most of them are working behind the scenes all over the world: Thailand, Eastern Europe, Brazil and other countries. Of course all energies are not created equal and all healers are not capable of transmitting energy of the highest caliber. If a healer has not cleared his or her own emotional issues, the transmission of energies will not be of the purest healing quality.

On a certain very popular cable news program, a neurosurgeon is employed as one of the medical consultants. One of the news commentators asked him why a very well-known female politician had a blood clot close to her brain. It was potentially very dangerous. He seemed unable to answer the question directly, which was embarrassing to watch as this learned man grasped for an answer. He obviously had no idea what causes blood clots. He talked about her history of having another blood clot in her leg and suggested she was prone to clotting. That might be true. But then why did she have the first clot over twenty years ago? I don't believe that having two clots twenty years apart is reason to believe she has a propensity for clotting.

Diseases are symbolic. They are the body's response to something that has gone wrong psychologically and emotionally in someone's life. Blood has to do with life force flow through the body. Obviously this person's life wasn't flowing as she would like it to. The treatment for clotting often includes using Coumadin to thin the blood and reduce the clot. It is actually rat poison. Again, I am not saying you shouldn't see a doctor when you are sick, but as you are likely aware, they ignore the real cause of disease, and the procedures they use are often very primitive.

A final story: I worked with a lady who had been diagnosed with skin cancer on her face. She was very attractive, had been a model, and greatly valued her appearance. When I talked to her on the phone, she said she had very little money and couldn't pay, so I said I would consider her situation and get back to her. I called her the next day and agreed to work with her. During our session, I transmitted healing energy to her. Two days later, she made an appointment with a doctor who surgically removed the growth on her face. The surgery left a dime-sized hole in her face to the right of her nose.

She was stunned by the appearance of the crater on her face. The biopsy showed that the tissue wasn't malignant. My personal belief is that it was malignant before I began working with her, but we will never know if it was actually cancer.

However, after the surgery the growth reappeared and became inflamed. She called me and asked to work with me again. We had five sessions, and after the sixth session she experienced a miraculous healing. The lesion on her face began to heal. Why was it so slow to heal in the beginning? Until she understood what it was trying to teach her, it would not heal. We had spent several sessions exploring the underlying issues and once she realized what they were, healing occurred.

I have explored and refined the use of energy healing and found the results to be spectacular. We are made of energy and it's no wonder that the cells of our bodies respond so positively to the stuff they are made of. For most people, healing life-threatening diseases like cancer, heart disease, and diabetes can become a crapshoot. All medical procedures treat symptoms only and do not get to the actual cause of the disease. When you truly understand how disease is created, you can begin to heal.

In this book, I have offered you a path to alternative healing that actually works. My sincere desire is that you will take this step on your journey to healing.

For further information or to contact Richard, you can find him in the following ways:

Email: richarddore@juno.com

Blog: www.selfempoweredhealing.blogspot.com

Acknowledgments

I would like to acknowledge and express my gratitude to the following people, for their support and contributions to the creation of this book:

Mary Carlson, for her tireless efforts, researching, typing, editing, and deciphering my handwriting. Without her perseverance and encouragement, this book would not exist.

Brooke Bennett, for her editing and careful attention to details.

Bruce Lipton, Ph.D., author of *The Biology of Belief,* who led me to a better understanding of modern biology and the role that mind and genes play in disease.

Eckhart Tolle, my spiritual teacher and author of *The Power of Now* and *A New Earth.*

Ann Meyer Makeever, author of *The Teaching of the Inner Christ,* for her contributions on The Law of Attraction.

Helen Schucman and William Thetford, for *A Course in Miracles.*

Harijiwan Khalsa, for sharing KundaliniYoga with the world.

Dr. David Clarke, my therapist of many years, for introducing me to spirituality.

Bob Fickes, a Vedic scholar, meditation master, and my meditation teacher.

Joan Solomon, who introduced me to rebirthing and the healing power of feelings.

Christian Mollitor and Adrienne Koch, Publisher and Managing Editor of Synclectic Media, for their enthusiasm in publishing this book.

And finally to all of my students, clients, and friends, who have been a source of inspiration throughout this writing project.

# # #